T0258079

# Contagion

DISEASE, GOVERNMENT, AND
THE "SOCIAL QUESTION" IN
NINETEENTH-CENTURY FRANCE

# CONTAGION

Disease, Government, and
the "Social Question" in
Nineteenth-Century France

ANDREW R. AISENBERG

Stanford University Press   Stanford, California

Stanford University Press
Stanford, California
© 1999 by the Board of Trustees of the
Leland Stanford Junior University
Printed in the United States of America
CIP data appear at the end of the book

# Acknowledgments

THIS BOOK BEGAN to take shape in the form of a dissertation completed under the supervision of John M. Merriman at Yale University. Throughout the long and challenging passage from dissertation to book, John has been unstinting in his offers of advice, information, and friendship. I want to acknowledge his long-standing support, and my own indebtedness to his blend of intelligence and love for France that makes him such a valued historian.

Many other colleagues, friends, and institutions have contributed to the completion of this book. I am grateful to the French government for a Bourse Chateaubriand and the Yale University Council on West European Studies for a dissertation research grant (with funds provided by the Mellon Foundation), both of which enabled me to undertake sustained research. In France, the staffs of the Bibliothèque Nationale, Archives Nationales, Archives de la Préfecture de Police de Paris, Bibliothèque Administrative de la Ville de Paris, Archives de la Ville de Paris et du Département de la Seine, Bibliothèque Interuniversitaire de Médecine, and the Bibliothèque Historique de la Ville de Paris made my research much easier. I want to extend special thanks to

Professor Alain Corbin, who took time to consider my project and to point me to crucial sources.

The bulk of the writing was completed in the United States in 1991 and 1992 at the School of Social Science, Institute for Advanced Study, Princeton. I want to thank Michael Walzer for inviting me to present an early version of chapter 4 at the school's Thursday Lunch Seminar, and Lucille Allsen and Meg Gilbert for making my stay there both productive and enjoyable. The European History Workshop at Stanford University, under the guidance of Paul Robinson, gave me another opportunity to present chapter 4 in 1993. Among the many individuals who read drafts of chapters, supplied useful information, and provided much needed intellectual and moral support along the way, I want to thank the following: Matthew Affron, Joshua Cole, the late Franco Ferraresi, Judy and Jerry Frank, Elisabetta Galeotti, Suzanne Greenberg, Kathy Kudlick, Mary Louise Roberts, Sophie Rosenfeld, and Debra Satz. Colin Jones and Sharon Marcus read the entire dissertation, and their comments helped immeasurably as I confronted the daunting task of transforming it into a book. In what I will always consider an exemplary act of friendship and collegiality, Sylvia Schafer read the completed manuscript, saving me from many errors in style and substance. It was my good fortune that Aron Rodrigue took an interest in this project; his keen intelligence, professional sense, and gift for friendship made all the difference.

The acknowledgment I most looked forward to offering is the one I now find the most difficult to express adequately. It was Joan Scott who first encouraged me to become a historian. Even after her official responsibilities as my undergraduate advisor at Brown ended, Joan never hesitated to support this project, helping me to articulate its structure, reading countless drafts, and offering editorial advice. I want to thank her especially for showing me the intellectual and political value of theoretically informed history writing, and for never doubting my ability to do it. I hope that this book approaches the very high standards she sets for her own work and that of her other students.

My family has endured the writing of this book for such a long time that I am afraid they will view an acknowledgment here as inadequate recompense. They know how grateful I am. My father died at a preliminary stage in the book's preparation. I wish he were here to see it completed; at the very least, I hope that it reflects the integrity he tried to impart to me. Finally, I could never have finished this book without Paul Klein's support and encouragement.

A.R.A.

# Contents

# Contagion

DISEASE, GOVERNMENT, AND
THE "SOCIAL QUESTION" IN
NINETEENTH-CENTURY FRANCE

# Introduction

THERE IS A CONSENSUS among historians about the importance of social reform for understanding France's most successful democratic experiment, the Third Republic. They disagree, however, in their interpretation of social reform and the light that it can shed on the operations of French democracy. For some historians, Third Republic social reform effected the fusion of political (formal) and socioeconomic (substantive) equality that had eluded earlier, unsuccessful Republican experiments. For others, the moralizing tenor of social reform betrayed its function as an instrument of social control that served to reconcile labor to its unequal position in a bourgeois social order rather than to create real equality. Different as they are, these two interpretative positions take the extension of "rights," the Revolutionary legacy of liberty and equality, as the foundation for late-nineteenth-century Republican social reform, and thus as the criterion by which to evaluate its successes, failures, and future potential in realizing a Republican social order.[1]

Recently, historians have offered a third interpretation that explains social reform as an attempt to surpass what contemporaries regarded as the delimiting Revolutionary categories of political liberty and equality—individual rights—in the establishment of a Republican social order.[2] These limitations, it is argued, first became manifest soon after the Revolution of February 1848, when an organized workers' movement sought to link the new Republic's support of universal political rights to "social rights"—that is, the government guarantee of consistent and fairly remunerated work. Their demand, and the inability of the provisional Republican government either to accept it or to find a suitable alternative solution to the problem of working-class unemployment and poverty, exposed the contradictions inherent in the category of rights. Intended to create a harmonious social order through the realization of political equality, the exercise of political rights ended up both depending upon and producing social distinctions. Workers expressed their understanding of this problem when they demanded, on behalf of a disenfranchised group, the recognition of their social equality as the necessary basis for exercising political rights. Nor could the category of rights offer government, whose mandate to protect the conditions of individual liberty was bound up with a respect for the inviolability of civil society and for the creation of free markets, a way of resolving the contradictory and politically volatile emergence of social inequality in a free industrial social order. Thus in June, the provisional Republican government violently repressed the workers' movement and the Republic itself was subsequently destroyed by Napoleon's 1851 coup d'état.[3]

Through the pursuit of social reform, so this interpretation goes, the Third Republic would confront the problematic relationship between rights and social order upon which its predecessor had foundered. It would do so, however, not by expanding the framework of political rights to include questions of substantive equality. Rather, social reform would reconceive the relationship of the individual to social order outside of the framework of individual rights, in the process providing government with the justifications and techniques to address the social problems and sources of social conflict created by the exercise of individual rights.

This book takes up this third interpretation by considering the regulation of contagious disease as a primary "site" where individualism, social order, and government in nineteenth-century Republican France were rearticulated.

IN WAYS BOTH REAL and metaphorical, contagion figured prominently in late-nineteenth-century social thought and policy. Republican politicians often cited the incidence of contagious disease among the working poor to support the government's obligation and capacity to eradicate the deleterious social problems associated with industrial life. They also invoked "contagion" to conjure up the social consequences of women's factory work and to justify the state's tutelary responsibility for "morally abandoned children."[4] Most important (and what made the preceding formulations possible), officials made contagion into the basis for objectifying the social ties and moral duties that bound together free individuals in a republic. In his formulation of "solidarism," the doctrinal justification for social reform developed by Third Republic politicians, Eugène d'Eichthal likened the organization of free individuals to an archipelago, islands linked by the bridges constituted through the "powerful currents of imitation or contagion."[5] Contagion manifested human interdependence as an integral part of the experience of individual liberty. It illustrated at once why autonomous individuals should care about one another and why government should intervene in social questions in addition to, and as part of, its larger task of protecting individual liberty.

Historians often trace this emphasis on contagion to Louis Pasteur, whose pathbreaking work on the microbial cause of epidemic diseases was coterminous with the establishment of the Third Republic in the last decades of the nineteenth century.[6] In doing so, they have largely reproduced the ways in which Third Republic scientists and government officials constructed the relationship between contagion and the possibilities of social reform. Such a connection was made forcefully by Paul Brouardel, a hygienist and dean of the Paris medical faculty well known both for his support of Pasteur and his efforts to establish a regulatory system of disease under the Third Republic. At the 1892 celebration of Pasteur's seventieth birthday held at the Sorbonne and attended by a host of Republican dignitaries, Brouardel waxed rhetorical: "Is it not you who have enabled doctors to demonstrate how one could preserve a city, a nation, a continent, from the most horrible scourges?"[7] For Brouardel, the scientific procedure that materialized a microbe in a laboratory culture effected a decisive break in how diseases would be understood and regulated. Before Pasteur, doctors and experimental scientists had offered "speculations" about disease, which at once referred to their supposed rejection of the explanatory category of contagion and the determining role of laissez-faire (noninterventionist) politics, not science, in that rejection. Henceforth, however, the rigor of scientific method would illuminate how diseases were spread in society and thus why Republican government was obliged to regulate them.

In light of recent historical research that has minimized the differences between Pasteurian advocates and their predecessors, it is worthwhile to ask why the official and scientific elite constructed such a rigid boundary between what did and did not constitute scientific explanations of disease.[8] True, Brouardel's early-nineteenth-century predecessors did not make the microbe the basis of their work. But their work often alluded to a role for a contagious agent that caused the spread of disease, and they stressed—again like their successors—the role of the insalubrious housing of the poor in the spread of diseases such as cholera, tuberculosis, and typhoid fever. Most important, however, these early-nineteenth-century hygienists did develop an understanding of the term "contagion." For them, it provided a basis for conceiving and regulating social problems without reference to the contested category of rights. By linking disease and poverty, contagion made the elimination of poverty neither a matter of recognizing the demands of the unruly poor upon government and society nor of limiting the rights of individuals or the operations of a free market. Rather, it imposed the duty of government to protect a social interest that transcended the interests and rights of individuals. Such a formulation of contagion was articulated early on by the July Monarchy hygienist Louis-René Villermé; once having located the causes of cholera in the insalubrious houses of the poor, he proceeded to expound on the moral contagion that operated in these hovels and that obliged government to moralize fathers, limit the factory work of mothers and wives, and remove children from a corrupting environment.[9]

It was precisely this removal of the possibility of social reform from the category of rights that led late-nineteenth-century scientists and officials to define earlier discussions about contagion outside the boundaries of science. For them, the explanation and regulation of the social causes of disease should illuminate the social duties that inhere in the exercise of political rights; in this way, the role of science in social reform would help realize the full potential of Republican liberty to address the social problems created by industrialization and urbanization. More often than not, they supported such a conviction by invoking scientific rationality. Science, because it was rooted in the faculty of human reason that also made possible the exercise of individual political rights, could inform only a government social agenda that took the Revolution's promise of liberty and equality as its goal.[10]

It is a testament to the staying power of these pronouncements linking scientific rationality and the Republican promise of liberty that historians unquestioningly accept the terms by which the late nineteenth century understood contagion and its place in a nascent Republican social-reform program.[11] Such pronouncements, however, efface certain characteristics that defined the regulation of contagious disease under the Third Republic. They do not explain how contagion came to define a social interest that transformed the most intimate aspects of the social life of free individuals—and especially the working poor—into an ongoing preoccupation of government. Nor do they explain why the attempt to control contagion found its ideal instrument not in the law—the guarantee of individual autonomy and limited government in a free society—but in an expanded police regulation that instituted government, rather than the rights-bearing individual, as "sovereign" in social matters. Finally, these terms fail to illuminate why the regulation of contagion defined the family, the recognized "site" of individual autonomy, as the pre-eminent locus of state intervention. These questions are best answered by resituating the possibilities of Pasteurian science, as an explanatory and regulatory system of both disease and social relations, in conceptions of contagion first proposed by hygienists in the 1830s and 1840s.

Why these early conceptions have been effaced, and what they might reveal about the relationship between contagion, science, and · social policy in nineteenth-century Republican France, cannot be explained as an instance of how the state misused science for the purposes of social control or for authoritarian ends. Rather, I want to emphasize the importance of these early formulations of contagion for understanding the discursive operations of science—and especially the human sciences such as medicine—that have constituted the possibilities of government in a free social order through a knowledge of the moral and social capacities of the "individual."

AS A DISCURSIVE PRACTICE, the human sciences took shape in the context of debates about democracy during the political crisis of late Old Regime France.[12] In the course of these debates, royal ministers with a reformist bent articulated their anxiety over the question of sovereignty. Confident in their rejection of a conception and practice of monarchical sovereignty that did not take the happiness of the people as its end, they nonetheless worried about whether the embrace of popular sovereignty would create social order. The human sciences offered a solution to this problem through a fractured understanding of the "individual."

On the one hand, the human sciences were based upon the contentions of John Locke, who claimed to have found in the exercise of senses and reason the human source of knowledge, freedom, and morality. True, the limitations of these faculties made a knowledge of only the social world possible; but it was precisely this limitation that imposed the individual as sovereign of society. In *An Essay Concerning Human Understanding* (1690), Locke made explicit how the definition of knowledge as an expression of human faculties was bound up with securing the moral capacities and interests of free individuals. He argued: "Our business here is not to know all things, but those which concern our conduct. If we can find out those measures whereby a rational creature, put in that state which man is in in this world, may and ought to govern his opinions and actions depending thereon, we need not be troubled that some other things escape our knowledge."[13] Human reason demonstrated knowledge, freedom, and morality as a single enterprise. Fostered by state institutions like the Academy of Sciences, the disciplines referred to collectively as a "Science of Man" became the focus of government ministers who recognized in human knowledge a powerful tool for reforming the structures of an absolutist monarchy and a hierarchical corporate society in accordance with the new value given to individual liberty and human happiness.

Under the auspices of state institutions, however, the human sciences transformed the individual into an object of investigation that ultimately served to express and address government concerns about the problems, and not the potentials, of human freedom.[14] If individual liberty might provide an antidote to the abuses of absolutism and the social hierarchy it simultaneously legitimized and depended upon, would the affirmation of human freedom lead to social order? Would the expression of a general political will, envisioned by Jean-Jacques Rousseau and accepted as the authoritative definition for democratic practice in eighteenth-century France, be a sociable one, a moral one?[15] In the context of these questions about the relationship between political liberty and social order, the human sciences came to define those specifically social capacities of human beings that were not produced by human reason and thus remained outside the realm of human freedom. Here, scientific rationality made the state, and not the individual, "responsible" for social order, a responsibility that would be realized through the cultivation of human morality and sociability. That science could serve as the basis for the social and moral authority of government in a free society without explicitly rejecting claims about individual liberty was due to the ambiguous status of reason. For if government justified its role in the making of a free social order by invoking the rational, and thus human, foundations of science, the definition and practice of scientific rationality (and thus the very definition of individualism and its relationship to social order) were always mediated by state interests and goals.

Medicine is an excellent example of this. Early in his short-lived public career, Louis XVI's controller general Anne-Robert-Jacques Turgot created the Royal Society of Medicine. Intended to address an epidemic that threatened French livestock, the society soon assumed as its responsibility the investigation and regulation of epidemics that afflicted humans as well. Through its preoccupation with these latter tasks, the society defined those social interests that, even in an order grounded in liberty, could not be left to individuals but required the intervention of the state. The causes of epidemics could be understood neither by individuals nor by local experts; a knowledge of their complex and variable "constitutions" required multiple sites of observation, assumed by state-appointed "epidemic doctors" and analyzed collectively by the Royal Society of Medicine. Nor could the treatment of epidemic diseases be left to individuals. If the society regarded epidemics as materializing the social bonds that tied individuals together, individuals—whether out of material self-interest (reluctance to slaughter contaminated cattle), ignorance (approaching a rabid pet dog), or shame (refusing to disinfect a contaminated house)—were either incapable of recognizing them as such or unwilling to do so. By requiring farmers to kill their cattle, by forcing families to take precautions against domestic animals and to disinfect their houses, the society would make the state responsible for informing individuals of their obligation to the health of the collective nation. In doing so, it defined the regulation of disease and the pursuit of health as central to the moral task of government that would transform the free individual into a "social man."[16]

It was not until the post-Thermidor period of the French Revolution, when politicians addressed the excesses of popular sovereignty displayed in the Terror as part of their attempt to "close" the Revolution, that medicine elaborated a role for government in the creation of a "social man." In a series of lectures given before the Section of Moral and Political Sciences at the recently established National Institute (the Royal Society of Medicine had been abolished along with other Old Regime corporate institutions, re-established only in 1820 by the Restoration Monarchy), Dr. P. J. G. Cabanis expounded on the "relations between the physical and the moral." Cabanis, whose work linked medicine, epistemology, and social reform, argued that differences in the physical characteristics of individuals (including, but not limited to, disease) accounted for the differential exercise of reason and morality. Early on, however, Cabanis's analysis moved from a consideration of the physical determinants of reason and morality to an exclusive focus on morality itself. If reason was the attribute of the free individual, morality was not an expression of reason (and thus not an attribute of the free individual). Rather, morality resulted from the interplay of physical variations and social circumstances. In Cabanis's analysis, the focus on physical differences served to separate the faculties of reason and morality, freedom and sociability. Reason is a uniform and universal attribute that makes political liberty and equality possible, while "the physical" is characterized by a variability that might account for differing patterns of sociability and formation of moral ideas that are manifested in human societies; reason marks the individual as autonomous and self-actualizing, while "the physical" shows individual moral capacity to be determined rather than determining. Cabanis developed this argument fully in his lecture on sexual difference, in which he attempted to demonstrate that women's physical constitution rendered them at once a source of morality and incapable of exercising those rational capacities that characterize free individuals. In the gap between the rational source of human freedom and the physical determinants of morality, the state becomes an indispensable force in a free social order. Through the scientific investigation and regulation of the physical and environmental determinants of morality, which Cabanis presents as the basis for a new, "philosophized" hygiene, the state asserts itself as responsible for transforming free individuals into sociable ones as well.[17]

Cabanis's definition of reason is crucial to understanding the discursive operations of science that constituted the social and moral authority of the state. For Cabanis does not address explicitly why the recognition of individual physical differences necessitates the separation of reason and morality. Nor does he explain why human reason is inadequate for making individuals both free and self-regulating, while scientific rationality makes the state ideally suited for assuming moral questions in a free society. His definition of reason becomes coherent only in relation to a vision of science as a source of legitimacy for the state in addressing the social problems and conflicts produced by democratic experience.[18]

IT IS AS AN EXPRESSION of Cabanis's vision of hygiene, and of the discursive operations of the Enlightenment "Science of Man" more generally, that this book will approach the nineteenth-century efforts to explain and regulate contagious disease in urban and industrial life. From Villermé in the July Monarchy to Paul Brouardel in the Third Republic, hygienists addressed the problem of disease under the auspices of state institutions, including (but not limited to) the Academy of Medicine, the Academy of Moral and Political Sciences (re-established in 1832, almost forty years after Napoleon had abolished it), and the ministerial Comité consultatif d'hygiène publique. Many of them matured intellectually, professionally, and politically as members of the Conseil de salubrité in the Department of the Seine (established by Napoleon I in 1802 and renamed the Conseil d'hygiène publique et de salubrité in 1851) and the journal *Annales d'hygiène publique*, a testament to the close association between national regulatory concerns and those of the capital that will be acknowledged in the pages that follow.[19]

Whatever the institutional context, however, hygienists displayed a keen, almost intuitive sense of the discursive operations of their discipline. They moved effortlessly back and forth between debates at the Academy of Medicine, where they proffered expert judgments about the role of the social life of the poor in the transmission of disease, and discussions at the Academy of Moral and Political Sciences, where they often invoked contagion to conjure up the dangers of (and thus the need to regulate) poverty and social conflict. In doing so, they materialized the process by which the problems of disease and poverty (as well as their own professional power) would be defined relationally. Hygienists appreciated how their pursuit of an effective regulation of disease would create new possibilities for government intervention in social life, possibilities that had been limited in the past by the Revolutionary principles of political and economic liberty but that were now rendered necessary by the emergence of social inequality and social conflict in a free society. Hygienists and their political allies consistently sought to realize this goal by including the regulation of disease in a broader project of social legislation. Their interest in legal regulation was not simply an attempt to apply the provisions of the 1790 Law on Municipalities and the Law of 12 Messidor An VIII (June 30, 1800, pertaining to the structure of government in Paris), which deemed epidemic disease a danger worthy of government intervention, to the problems of contagion in the nineteenth century. More important, hygienists recognized how those foundational laws dating from the Revolution objectified disease as one of those infrequent yet serious dangers in social life (along with fires and revolutions) through which the intermittent and repressive function of government in a free society would be conceived. Through their own scientific understanding of the danger posed by disease, hygienists sought nothing less than to transform the extent and mechanisms of legal government intervention in social life.

These connections between science and government regulation of the social are best viewed by considering the enduring presence, both before and after Pasteur's investigations, of the working-class dwelling in the attempts to explain and regulate contagious disease.[20] A decontextualized epistemology of science—one that defines science and politics as independent if occasionally collaborative endeavors—cannot account for why hygienists favored the dwelling over other, equally valid factors in their attempts to explain and regulate disease. To explain this sustained interest in the working-class dwelling requires that we acknowledge the relevance of the political resonance of the "home" in the production of scientific understandings of disease. In French Republican discourse, the home constituted the moral capacities of self-regulating individuals that would establish liberty, and not government, as a source of social order. By associating disease with the space and function of the home, hygienists transformed morality from an attribute of the free individual to a task of government, necessary for addressing the social problems produced in urban and industrial social life.

My own appreciation of the multiple and interrelated meanings of the home that linked the scientific project of disease regulation to the political one of social regulation has been shaped significantly by recent studies emphasizing the gendered and familial terms of nineteenth-century social reform.[21] These studies have argued convincingly that government officials created new justifications and techniques for intervention in social life by defining industrial social problems as moral problems pertaining, above all, to the functions of sexual difference and family organization. Such a recourse to sexual difference and the family dissociated the faculty and expression of morality from individual liberty and thus made social suffering and social conflict accessible to government regulation. This book is, in part, an attempt to both confirm and complement those studies by demonstrating how definitions of morality in terms of sexual difference were constituted through science. It was the universalistic truth claims of science that made such a paradoxical recourse to sexual difference as the source of morality appear both convincing and natural. In turn (and this is the major point of the pages that follow), such references to truth and universalism in realizing government regulation of morality expose the discursive operations of science.

This examination of the place of contagion in the development of nineteenth-century social regulation is organized chronologically and analytically. This book begins chronologically, in Chapter 1, with early understandings of contagion and attempts to regulate contagious disease in the 1830s and 1840s, decades defined by two cholera epidemics and escalating social conflict. Chapter 2 proceeds to chart the innovative Second Republic and Second Empire experiments in government (including but not limited to "Haussmannization") that brought together disease regulation and social regulation. Chapter 3 charts the debate over contagion that emerged around Pasteur's controversial "theory of germs" in the late 1870s and 1880s. The book concludes in Chapters 4 and 5 with the efforts of Third Republic politicians to create new regulatory institutions and techniques for preventing disease and to solidify them through the passage of a public health law in 1902.

The organization of the book also offers a framework for understanding the role of contagion in social regulation discursively—that is, for exploring the links between knowledge about disease and government intervention in social life in a way that emphasizes the interrelations of "political" and "scientific" factors and interests. To this end, the first two chapters investigate how government concerns about understanding and regulating the problems of disease and poverty came together in the fashioning of the category of contagion in the 1830s and 1840s. Chapters 3, 4, and 5 attempt to show how this conception of contagion, and the complex of government regulatory interests it expressed, shaped late-nineteenth-century "Pasteurian" science and regulation. These latter chapters begin by posing the ambiguous and open-ended character of Pasteur's contributions to disease explanation and regulation, and then proceed to analyze the heterogeneous, sometimes inchoate and contested, professional and political interests (such as conflicts between hygienists and engineers and rivalries between different administrative authorities, debates over the causes of poverty, and questions about government intervention in the home and the role of the law in regulation) that structured the debate over contagion, and that ultimately enabled specific understandings of contagion and regulatory practices to eclipse others.

Throughout the narrative, I will employ textual analysis, paying close attention to the language of scientists, hygienists, government administrators, and politicians for the links between scientific and political considerations in the formulation of a knowledge about contagion. My intention here is not to reduce the biological reality of disease, or a scientific knowledge of disease, to "words." Rather, I have found attention to language helpful in materializing the complex process by which scientific explanations of disease, professional identities, and government capacities were defined relationally.

Nor is such an approach meant to deny the benefits of scientific progress or the effectiveness of public health laws. Indeed, it is because these questions have dominated previous historical studies of contagion that they do not occupy a prominent position in this book.[22] More important, however, I believe that a discursive analysis that materializes the political and professional determinants of scientific knowledge about contagion will provide a more complex and satisfying historical account of why disease received then—as it does now—so much attention and generated so much heated debate in official circles. A discursive approach will also provide a much needed rethinking of the transformation of Republicanism in its encounter with the painful and unintended social consequences associated with industrialization and urbanization. At the heart of this transformation was an expanded conception and practice of government that was not premised upon a natural and incontestable reality of a free individual, but rather that was created through new ways of thinking about individuals and their relationship to society.

## CHAPTER I

# Contagious Poverty

## Introduction: The Cholera Epidemic of 1832

Cholera reached Paris in the spring of 1832.[1] To a certain extent, government officials in charge of regulating epidemic disease were prepared for its arrival. Cholera was first reported in Bengal in 1826. Upon its spread westward to Moscow (1830) and Poland (1831), the state Academies of Sciences and Medicine sent commissions there to investigate the epidemiology of the disease, and more specifically to determine whether it was contagious (spread by an agent through human contact) or infectious (produced by banal factors present in the urban environment). Back at home, the ministry of the interior instructed prefects, the state-appointed governors of departments, to organize regulatory commissions and implement precautions. In Paris, the prefecture of police empowered a Cholera Commission to be formed under the aegis of the departmental (prefectoral) Conseil de salubrité.

The conseil had been established in 1802 to investigate and regulate instances of "insalubriousness" in Paris and its environs. In this endeavor, the conseil implemented the provisions of existing legislation, which gave priority to Old Regime definitions and sites of insalubriousness that indicted the dangerous infectious smells ("miasmas") in urban surroundings; rotting garbage and excrement in streets and sewers, cemeteries, and prostitution were just a few of the concerns that preoccupied conseil members in the fulfillment of their duties here. In addition, new dangers associated with an urbanizing and industrializing capital began to preoccupy the conseil, such as "hazardous" industries emerging in the center of Paris and food quality control.[2]

The threat of cholera promised to intensify and transform the activity of the conseil, which anticipated new needs by creating a network of twelve arrondissement and forty-eight neighborhood commissions composed of doctors, pharmacists, local notables, and supervised by arrondissement mayors and local police officers. In 1831, well before the epidemic reached Paris, these commissions investigated, and proposed regulations for, unhealthful and dirty conditions in Paris that might facilitate the spread of disease. The commission that oversaw the Left Bank neighborhood surrounding the Luxembourg palace alone investigated over nine hundred potential trouble spots—including public spaces, industrial buildings, and dwellings—and made more than four hundred recommendations for sanitary improvements; the prefect of police received a total of ten thousand reports from neighborhood commissions.[3]

But it would have been impossible to prepare for the shock of cholera. The disease attacked the population in a hard and quick manner, especially in Paris. Cholera produced abundant diarrhea and vomiting in its victims, often leading to death by dehydration within forty-eight hours. At the height of the epidemic in March and April, when cholera killed more than eight hundred Parisians a day, both the Hôtel Dieu and Necker hospitals were full. The Charité had only twelve available beds. By the end of 1832, one out of every eighteen inhabitants had contracted the disease, and more than eighteen thousand of them had died.[4]

The challenge to explain and regulate this violent, unfamiliar disease was complicated by the threat of social conflict in the capital and other industrial centers in France. Beginning in the 1830s, workers organized to protest the transformations in work that characterized early industrial capitalism—competition, subcontracting, cyclical unemployment, and wage cuts. The stage for this social conflict was set by Louis-Philippe, the July Monarch who ascended to power in 1830 as the protector of individual political liberty but who, in the view of an organized workers' movement, colluded with selfish industrialists against the working poor.[5] The disproportionate number of workers and poor among the victims of cholera suggested to them the continuation of the war against labor by other than economic means. The suspicion that government officials were poisoning workers with cholera intensified the popular impression of the hospital as the place where one goes to die, and workers often refused the care offered there by doctors.[6] In April of 1832, workers participated in "cholera riots," killing as many as five suspected poisoners. Among the victims were an employee of the ministry of the interior suspected of having spread poison in a wine shop and two sweet merchants accused of selling poisoned candy to children near the Place de la Grève, where unemployed workers waited, often in vain, for offers of employment. In June, the funeral of the popular Napoleonic general Lamarque, attended by twenty-four thousand spectators and ten thousand troops, occasioned two days of street fighting that began when someone fired a shot into the crowd of mourners. As in the case of the "cholera riots," the fighting took place in established areas of popular militancy in the central and eastern neighborhoods of the Right Bank: St. Antoine, St. Denis, St. Martin, and St. Méry.[7]

The "social question"—how to address the problems of poverty and social conflict—would figure prominently in the attempts of official administrators and scientists to explain and regulate cholera. The relationship between cholera and the social question, however, cannot be adequately explained in terms of what are often taken to be the opposing categories of "science" and "politics." The cholera epidemic of 1832 arrived on the heels of a significant, if highly contested, moment in the making of modern medical science: the advent of physiological medicine.[8] Physiological medicine took as its premise the idea that disease is an expression of human physiological laws; its aim was to discover, explain, and regulate the conditions that cause the laws governing human life to produce morbid expressions. In defining disease as a product of human life, physiological medicine revealed its relationship to the larger Enlightenment project of the "Science of Man." For to define disease in terms of human physiological laws was to deny the traditional ontological status of disease, a phenomenon that, often described as an "evil," was both foreign to human experience and inaccessible to the explanatory powers of human reason. Now the study of disease would contribute to a larger appreciation and understanding of humanity, while the investigation and control of the conditions that caused physiological laws to go "awry" would realize the capacity of science to contribute to human perfection and happiness. From its very inception at the beginning of the nineteenth century, however, the potential of physiological medicine was limited by what appeared to be an insurmountable problem: how to reconcile a search for the determining causes of physiological laws and their capacity for morbid expressions with a conception of the "individual," so central to Enlightenment thought, as an autonomous, self-regulating being. The articulation of this contradiction manifested the political constitution of the discipline of physiological medicine and the larger enterprise of a Science of Man, for the deterministic vision of human life as governed by laws made human potential dependent upon the regulatory practices and institutions of science, which in France were bound up with state power. But how could science (and by, implication, the state), which was itself regarded as an expression of the rationality that defined human beings as self-regulating and that took as its object the happiness of free individuals, pose the "individual" as determined and thus an object of regulation?[9]

It was the recognition of this contradiction, and the difficulty of resolving it, that accounts for the numerous and different ways physiologists and pathologists conceived the laws of life and disease: from Xavier Bichat's famous anatomical observations (undertaken during the Revolution) of the lesions produced by the laws governing tissual systems, to François Broussais's understanding of disease as an expression of the capacity of the tissues for inflammation (the decade beginning in 1810 and the 1820s), to Claude Bernard's experimental demonstration of disease as a product of the chemical (nutritive) properties contained in the tissues (1840s to 1860s). Different as they were, however, each of these contributions to physiological medicine was characterized by convoluted formulations, consistently (and unsuccessfully) aimed at reconciling an understanding of life as determined by laws with the conception of the self-regulating individual. Bichat divided the laws that governed the body's nineteen tissual systems into two categories: physical (held in common with other phenomena, constant, and thus accessible to observation and explanation) and vital (unique to human beings, variable, and thus inexplicable). Bichat also presented the specific diseases that characterized the different tissual systems as the product of interchangeable banal causes, or worse yet, as simply inexplicable. Bernard attempted to offset the determinism that grounded his understanding of tissual properties by acknowledging the *"individualité effroyable"* (which he also referred to as "idiosyncrasy") and indeterminacy of human life. He found this individuality and indeterminacy manifested, above all, in the *"milieu intérieur,"* the product of the capacity of the tissual properties contained in the organs to create the very chemical conditions of their own life.[10]

In official debates about explaining and regulating cholera, references to contagion often expressed the potential and problems, at once scientific and political, of physiological medicine. The category of contagion, in a more stark manner than its popular rival "infection," presumed a cause for disease and thus brought to the fore the conflict between the determinism of life and disease and the self-determining attribute of physiological laws. This conflict became particularly acute when investigators who entertained the possibility of a contagious cause for cholera could not satisfactorily explain the problems of differential reception and variable transmission. The willingness of respected scientists to support contagion or infection, and the authoritative, if not always convincing, evidence that could be marshaled in support of either position, only exposed the imprecision of the category "contagion" and the larger structural problems of physiological medicine, leading one 1832 report to conclude that "[in] their writings not all doctors have given the same meaning to the word contagion . . . often argu[ing] over words without much use to science."[11] In the end, the only clear conclusion that could be drawn from this debate over the relative merits of contagion and infection was the challenge it posed for the future of physiological medicine: "to understand the theoretical implications of these new observations of cholera."[12]

The conundrum of differential reception and variable transmission was often reduced to the question of why the poor suffered disproportionately during the epidemic. As such, the efforts to ascertain whether cholera was a contagious or infectious disease could not avoid a second and equally difficult question about the appropriate role of government in social life that was at the heart of physiological medicine and the larger project of the Science of Man. Ironically, in the context of a seemingly irresolvable debate between contagion and infection, contagion ended up finding its clearest formulation in expressions of social fear. Contagion invoked anxiety about the repressive tendencies of government that sometimes accompanied disease regulation. Here, the previous Restoration government provided a frightening example of what might occur. In an attempt to prevent the spread of yellow fever over the Franco-Spanish border, the government had secured the passage of a sanitary law in 1822 that included quarantines on land and in ports (thus severely restricting commerce) and the death penalty for those who transgressed the law and facilitated contagion.[13] Contagion also figured prominently in the workers' suspicion of a government-orchestrated cholera plot, while the city's wealthier residents (some of whom fled the site of the epidemic) invoked contagion to conjure up the multiple dangers posed by the sick and unruly laboring poor.

When in 1832, after the epidemic had subsided, the minister of the interior established a second cholera commission to explain the deadly epidemic that earlier had eluded them, contagion would become indispensable to the "theoretical" evaluation of physiological medicine. Through contagion, the scientific explanation of cholera, and especially why it favored the poor, would provide new ways of thinking about and regulating social problems without referring to the category of the autonomous, self-regulating individual.

## The Cholera Commission Report of 1834

Neither the category of contagion, nor the lofty scientific and political issues it was intended to address, were immediately evident. To the contrary, the Cholera Commission prefaced the findings contained in its 1834 report in surprisingly modest, even negative terms. It sought to avoid any consideration of the contested questions of science and politics that had linked the epidemic to the escalation of social and political conflict in the capital. Composed largely of the same bureaucrats, notables, doctors, and (most important) hygienists who had heeded the ministry's call on the eve of the epidemic two years earlier, the commission intended to realize the objective of this second task by refusing to make the category of contagion the basis of its investigation.[14]

Instead, the commission pursued its task by analyzing the conditions that facilitated cholera. Conditions were a category tied to the emergence of a neo-Hippocratic "environmentalism" in the eighteenth century. It became identified with the efforts of hygienists to detect and eliminate disease-causing miasmas produced by influences that were topographical ("exhalations of the earth"), demographic (sex, age), moral (excess), and social (badly constructed or humid buildings). Conditions were, by definition and in practice, a flexible and expandable category. If hygienists took that category seriously as the basis for their enhanced authority and expertise since the end of the eighteenth century, others (most notably physiologists and pathologists) questioned its scientific status, especially when considered in relation to the Newtonian category of cause that informed the aspirations of a nascent physiological medicine. Both Bichat and Bernard appreciated the hygienist's knowledge of the conditions implicated in the production of disease, but only because the primary causes that made physiological laws produce morbid symptoms remained elusive.[15] Indeed, it was precisely such a secondary status, as a category that expressed the ancillary influences upon disease, that led commission members to adopt conditions as the basis for their investigations. For a reliance upon "conditions" would allow them at least to suggest a tentative explanation and regulations for cholera without broaching the (scientifically and politically) charged category of "cause."

But the commission's reliance upon the category of "conditions" possessed other meanings and usages. It drew upon Cabanis's reformulation of hygiene as a "Science of Man" that henceforth would focus on the interplay of physical and environmental circumstances that determined the different moral capacities of individuals. Cabanis's influence here revealed the intent of the commission as not to avoid the endeavors of science and government altogether, but rather to reject a vision of their relationship which took as its basis and goal the rational and autonomous individual. Through this focus on the conditions that produced cholera, and especially why the poor predominated among its victims, the report would provide a new way to understand and regulate poverty.

These two usages of conditions shaped the trajectory of the commission's investigation of cholera. The report began by considering those unhealthy conditions that had preoccupied the efforts of an increasingly ubiquitous hygiene movement in the years immediately preceding the cholera epidemic: the role of topography, of climate, of the density and height of buildings, and of sex and age. But the analysis of these established understandings of conditions failed to explain why cholera was deadly in Paris, or why some individuals got sick while others did not. What especially surprised the commission was that some of the urban spaces that hygienists had long decried as dangerous exhibited lower rates of cholera than other neighborhoods of Paris renowned for their cleanliness. In particular, the report noted the comparatively benign influence exerted upon the population by the notorious garbage dump of Montfauçon—that "epicenter of stench in Paris,"[16] full of rotting horse carcasses—and the commune of Gentilly traversed by the polluted Bièvre River.

Faced with these setbacks, the report moved to a consideration of the role of poverty in the spread of cholera, defined here as the "*conditions d'existence*" of the poor: what kind of work they did, where they lived, and, most important, *how* they lived.[17] This move might seem both abrupt and surprising, given that a debate about the meaning of poverty was at the center of growing social conflict in the 1830s. Reformers and industrialists, often under the auspices of government institutions, argued that poverty resulted from immoral behavior. In a society that had recently embraced the principle of individual liberty and equality, they concluded, only workers, and not the state, could be held "responsible" for their poverty. An increasingly organized and vocal workers' movement regarded poverty as the product of the unjust operations of a free market that deprived workers of their rights to liberty and equality. Consequently, they demanded that the state, in its role as the protector of liberty, regulate the problem of poverty by securing for workers their "social rights" to steady work and a living wage. The incommensurate understandings of rights that fueled the debate between workers and the alliance of industrialists and politicians gave expression to the paradox of the Revolutionary legacy of rights. For late-eighteenth-century political theorists and Revolutionary actors, the recognition and exercise of rights would serve to establish a new social order grounded in the political equality of free individuals, without any reference to the social distinctions that defined the hierarchical society of Old Regime France. But the emergence of poverty in the nineteenth century implicated the exercise of rights in the creation of new social distinctions and, in turn, revealed how social distinctions determined access to the exercise of political rights. As such, the debate over poverty put into question whether the Revolutionary legacy of individual political rights could create a free social order.[18]

In presenting the *conditions d'existence* as an explanation for cholera, the commission members revealed how thoroughly they had associated the need to explain and regulate the problems of cholera and poverty. The report invoked "disorder" to signify, and thus bring together, the scientific question of why the poor predominated among its victims and the political problem of working-class poverty and militancy. "[I]n observing these frequent contradictions, these consistently variable relations [in the appearance of cholera]," the report stated, "the commission has not been able to prevent itself from suspecting in this disorder that it sees everywhere the existence of an ever-present disturbance, and from believing that this [disturbance] can only be the population itself. . . ."[19] In the end, the report devised the category of *conditions d'existence* of the poor as much to resolve the political problem of poverty as to explain cholera. For to define poverty as a condition of cholera was to remove a consideration of poverty from the contested category of rights, and thus to approach it as an object that even a government normally restricted in its power by individual political rights could and should regulate.

The manner in which "conditions" denied a relationship between poverty and rights, and thus provided a new way of conceiving and regulating social problems, was made evident in the report's analysis of that most valued social activity, work. Enlightenment philosophes had considered work as the endeavor that fostered and illuminated the moral capacities of free, rights-bearing individuals. The organized workers' movement drew upon this conception when demanding that government, in the interest of individual rights and dignity, provide steady and fairly remunerated employment that had been deprived them by rapacious industrialists, even if such a guarantee meant intervening in the free operations of the market.[20] But the report's consideration of work as a condition in the transmission of cholera avoided a representation of that activity as an expression of the attributes of free and sociable individuals. Instead, and following from the definition of conditions offered at the outset, the report objectified work as a determining factor—is work performed inside or outside? while sitting down or standing up? in a ventilated or unventilated workshop?[21]

But perhaps more indicative of the report's intent to have an explanation of cholera serve as the basis for an understanding of poverty that would avoid the conflict between political (formal) and substantive (social) rights was the way in which it ended up minimizing the importance of work. For no matter how considerable the influence of work on disease appeared to be, individuals presented specific habits—"*moeurs et habitudes*"[22]—that mediated its role in the production of cholera. This category included numerous and variable "excesses" such as drinking, diet, and fatigue that made analysis difficult. The report nevertheless did find a way to explain these individual influences on cholera, and thereby to avoid the potential obstacle their variability posed to explanation, by associating them with the working-class dwelling. The report stated: "There exists a certain kind of population [the poor], like a certain kind of place [the dwelling of the poor], which favors the development of cholera, rendering it more intense and its effects more lethal."[23] Here, "like" ["comme"] specifies the poor's "way of life" ["*genre de vie*"] alongside the dwelling as a condition that favored the transmission of cholera; it also suggests that their "way of life" is "like" the dwelling space. This comparison contributed to the goal of explaining and regulating cholera by organizing the diverse moral influences on cholera in one space—the dwelling—and by transforming morality, in accordance with the category of "conditions," into a determined phenomenon.[24] The focus on the dwelling as the source of the moral causes of cholera also ensured that the explanation of cholera would provide a new understanding of poverty. It did so not simply by favoring a moral interpretation of poverty over an economic one, but also by avoiding references to the capacities of the autonomous individual altogether. The immorality of the poor, by virtue of the danger that it posed in propagating disease and the scientific expertise needed to illuminate its spatial determinants, provided a compelling social interest and new techniques for government to regulate poverty. Thus the report concluded:

[N]o one will doubt that the habits [*habitudes*], customs [*moeurs*], and the existence of a large segment of its population are to be considered important [in this matter]. . . . [T]here exists in our midst a numerous class which is forced to subsist by means of onerous [*pénible*] work, and to which the solicitude of the government must be extended at all times to protect [this class] from those dangers which it cannot or does not know how to combat. . . .

Besides, no matter how depraved this population may be, it is not the place of the commission to judge its morals.// There is a truth that it is necessary to repeat lest one forget it, that there exist between the person [*l'homme*] and his surroundings secret bonds, mysterious relations, whose influence on him is constant and deep. Favorable, this influence fortifies his physical and moral forces, it develops and conserves those forces[;] harmful, it alters them, destroys them, kills them. But its action is never to be feared more [than] when it manifests itself in a crowded population.[25]

For the members of the commission, the policy implications of the state's new social responsibility to regulate working-class morality were clear: Clean up the housing of the poor and build new housing.

Hygienists, philanthropists, and some government officials had un-successfully advocated such a policy before the cholera epidemic. The possible return of cholera, however, rendered necessary a governmental intervention in what was once considered to be a contractual matter between two free individuals, the landlord and the tenant. Thus, the report warned: "The influence of the aforementioned causes would become deadly if epidemic or contagious diseases were to develop in the capital."[26]

In the end, then, the focus on the conditions of the dwelling of the poor brought the report back to the terrain of contagion that, at the outset, it had claimed to avoid. The home resolved the two problems that had placed an acceptance of contagion at odds with the possibility of a medical explanation of cholera. One could now invoke contagion without having to resolve the tension between cause and physiological laws in the production of disease; the contagious cause was always mediated by, indeed inseparable from, the domestic environment that served as the "envelope" of the body.[27] This merging of the contagious agent and the body's physiological laws in the conditions of the home explained why the poor might have been more likely to contract cholera. The conditions of the working-class home also demonstrate how important the political question of working-class poverty and militancy was for the re-emergence of contagion in a medical explanation of cholera. Those conditions of the home that indicted the moral practices of the poor in the production of cholera also explained why a state limited in its regulatory capacities by the principle of individual liberty was nonetheless obliged to regulate immorality as the cause of poverty. Now defined as the cause of disease, the morality of the poor had become socialized.

### Villermé

Nowhere was the mutual constitution of the explanations of cholera and poverty more readily apparent than in the emergence of contagion as a category of social analysis. Contagion figured prominently in the first major social investigation of the Academy of Moral and Political Sciences. In 1834, the year of the publication of the Cholera

Commission's report, the academy charged two of its members who had also served on the commission, the influential hygienist Louis Villermé and the doctor and social investigator Louis François Benoiston de Chateauneuf, to investigate the "physical and moral conditions" of workers in the textile trades, the leading sector of industrial production in early-nineteenth-century France. Only Villermé's contribution was published, in 1840, as *Tableau de l'état physique et moral des ouvriers employés dans les manufactures de coton, de laine et de soie.*

In 1832, soon after he ascended to the throne, the liberal "July Monarch" Louis Philippe had re-established the Academy of Moral and Political Sciences.[28] The academy had served briefly (as the Second Section of the National Institute) under the Directory as a forum that would place scientific investigation in the service of the state's attempt to understand and resolve a wide variety of social problems. As the first major commission of the reconstituted academy, the investigation of the textile industries demonstrated how profoundly the problems of working-class poverty and militancy shaped the July Monarchy's interest in pursuing the relationship between science and government. The year 1834 was one of intense labor agitation in industrial France, which culminated in April with the Lyon silkworkers' uprising. Members of this elite segment of the textile industry, confronted with the de-skilling of their craft, unemployment, and wage cuts that characterized the advent of industrial capitalism in France, took to the streets and demanded their "social rights," vowing to "Live Working or Die Fighting."[29]

Villermé had the radical social demands and militant methods of the Lyon silkworkers in mind when he defended (hygienic) science as an ideal and necessary approach for resolving the problem of poverty that beset the burgeoning textile industries.[30] In his view, the "scrupulous exactitude" of this science would dissipate the erroneous explanations and proposed remedies for poverty in terms of rights that "party politics" had "spread" among workers.[31] To that end, Villermé focused on the question of wages. The workers' movement had made this question central to its critique of industrial capitalism. The question of wages did not signify a preoccupation with material deprivation (although this was certainly relevant). Rather, for workers it promised to reveal the contradictions of industrial liberty that had promoted the prosperity of industrialists by depriving artisans of their rights to steady work and a living wage.

But Villermé asked a different question about wages. Through a scientific study, he sought to determine whether workers in the textile and silk industries could live on the wages they earned. He sought an answer to that question by shifting the focus of analysis away from the structure of industrial production and markets to what had served as the basis of the Cholera Commission report: the family and the *conditions d'existence* of its members. Villermé calculated and compared average wages and living expenses for different branches of the textile trades in different regions of the country, taking into account the wage contributions and living expenses of the male head of household and other family members. He concluded that cyclical unemployment made subsistence difficult for many working-class families. But, he continued, families that embraced sobriety and thrift and in which the wife and mother supplemented her husband's salary *and* raised her children by taking in piecework could survive what, for those families composed of drunkards, spendthrifts, and absent working mothers, were devastating industrial crises. As evidence of the determining role of working-class immorality in poverty, Villermé presented evidence of the tragic plight of families in which parents and their four children shared a single bed, husbands and fathers wasted their time and money at the cabaret, mothers and wives indulged their taste for "*la toilette*," and children worked at an age when their only preoccupation should have been games.

Informed as it was by the category of conditions that resulted from the investigation of cholera, Villermé's indictment of these moral causes did not lead him to advocate workers' responsibility for their own poverty. Instead, conditions enabled him to avoid the politically contested category of individualism altogether, and to offer instead a vision of working-class immorality that, now associated with the cause and spread of disease, required government intervention as the solution to the problem of poverty. In order to convince his audience of academy members and government officials of their obligation to address the problem of poverty through the regulation of working-class morality, Villermé began by offering compelling evidence of the role of immorality in disease. "No illness is associated exclusively with specific industrial workplaces," he argued, "but there are some diseases which appear more frequently when the living conditions of workers favor their development."[32] Thus, Villermé alluded to mothers who, because they accepted industrial work in factories and hired wet nurses to care for their infants, ended up with scrofulous children. He also noted that in the Lorraine town of Ste.-Marie-Aux-Mines, weavers who lived in crowded dwellings near the factory appeared to be in bad health, in stark contrast to agricultural workers nearby who appeared "so fresh, so ruddy."[33]

This presentation of the moral causes of disease led Villermé next to define immorality itself as a disease that eventually led to poverty:

> Thus incivility, immorality, bad inclinations, deprivation, and poverty are transmitted from generation to generation by the force of a contagious example, and are perpetuated by the force of habit, just as good morals and qualities are perpetuated among other classes and other workers, or even among workers from the same classes who inhabit different lodgings.[34]

Here, the metaphor of contagion facilitated Villermé's transition from a consideration of the moral causes of disease among workers to an understanding of working-class poverty as a moral pathology. The historian of science James Bono has argued recently that metaphors serve as a "link" between scientific and political discourses, thereby illuminating "the constitution of scientific discourses as synchronic systems of meaning within a constellation of other cultural and social systems."[35] In Villermé's analysis, the metaphor of contagion provided a link between the explanations of disease and poverty that was informed by the imperative of government regulation. The moral causes of disease offered two crucial criteria that invalidated the category of the autonomous individual as the basis for understanding and regulating poverty and that, instead, imposed the necessity of state regulation: It presented working-class immorality as a threat to society, and it made the perception of that threat dependent on scientific expertise. For Villermé, then, the definition of poverty as a moral disease led him to advocate a government regulation of the working poor, a regulation that because it addressed these moral concerns through the family would not require the July Monarchy to reject its commitment to industrial liberty. Thus he concluded: "[R]emove [*arracher*] infants and children from the contagious examples of intemperance and immorality that the parents provide. . . . [A]ll of those measures that do not aim at removing them from their [parents'] pernicious influence will allow the disease to spread."[36] In the end, hygienic "objectivity," contrary to what Villermé argued at the beginning of his investigation, did not banish politics from the analysis of poverty; rather, it constituted a new form of state social politics.

Sexual difference was central to Villermé's elaboration of this politics.[37] As the above passages suggest, his vision of the moral agency of the state took women and children as its exclusive object. As in so many other aspects of his argument, Villermé relied upon references to disease in order to develop a moral regulation of poverty that preoccupied, above all, the lives of women and children. Villermé consistently minimized the relationship between industrial work and the incidence of disease among men; for to admit the validity of such an assertion, often proposed by the workers' movement, would be to endorse an understanding of social inequality as a product of industrial liberty, and thus of the contradictions inherent in the conception and implementation of "rights." But Villermé did not demonstrate such reticence when it came to discussing the incidence of disease among female industrial workers. He argued that the capitalist transformation of those trades, especially the mechanization of certain aspects of production and the manufacturer's overriding concern with profits, had made women an ideal (because unskilled and thus cheap) source of labor. Their assumption of work, however, had increased their chances of contracting consumption.[38] Thus, he took issue with the generalizations about work and disease put forward by Dr. Patissier in his 1822 *Traité des maladies des artisans*:

My investigations do not confirm what he has said about varicose veins and ulcers on the legs, and neither have I observed that carders, spinners, shearers, and teaselers suffer more than others from pulmonary afflictions. I have only seen [that] women and children employed as carders are quite often more pale than other workers of the same sex and age.[39]

In those cases where the evidence of disease among male workers appeared incontrovertible, Villermé indicted the practices of industrial capitalism only indirectly, accounting for them as the result of the same unfavorable "living conditions"—quality of lodging, fatigue, diet, clothing, and *moeurs*—that resulted when women abandoned their family for industrial work. In either scenario, women's new position in factory production constituted the moral source of disease and poverty. Not only did it make them sick but their assumption of factory work also led them to neglect their role as wives and mothers, resulting in the spread of disease and poverty to their family members. Thus he observed with dismay those working mothers who "some days could only breast feed their children during the few short hours they spent at home,"[40] certain proof, in his view, of why so many infants in industrial cities contracted scrofula.

Villermé employed this evidence of the relationship between disease and women's industrial work to make moral pronouncements and offer a social agenda on behalf of the state that was directed exclusively at women. He argued that women should be restricted from accepting factory work; instead they should return to the family and resume their domestic duties as wives and mothers, which would also allow them to accept piecework as a way of supplementing the husband's precarious wage. At the same time, however, Villermé rejected the possibility of regulating men's factory work, which, in his view, would infringe upon industrial liberty. To justify this government intervention, however restricted, in the industrial workplace as well as his call for the (more expansive) regulation of working-class family life, Villermé defined the pernicious moral consequences of women's industrial work—mixed-sex workshops, serial relationships, and prostitution—as contagious.

Villermé's association of contagion and women demonstrates

how the scientific understanding of the moral causes of disease among the poor was defined in relation to a larger project of government regulation in a free industrial social order. In positing that association, Villermé demonstrated his indebtedness to the founder of modern hygiene, Cabanis. From the lectern of the academy's predecessor (the Second Section of the institute) some forty years earlier, Cabanis had presented scientific evidence of morality as a function of women's physical difference. In doing so, Cabanis rearticulated the relationship between reason and morality that had grounded the Enlightenment belief in the self-regulating capacities of free individuals. Women's physical difference not only defined their moral capacities; it also deprived them of the reason that made possible the exercise of political liberty. As a function now determined by "the physical" rather than by human reason, the operations of morality could be known and realized only through scientific rationality, which (as Cabanis's own presentation before the institute amply demonstrated) was bound up with state power and institutions. To be sure, the way in which Cabanis and Villermé conceived of the relationship between "the moral and physical" was vastly different, a result of the momentous events that transformed France in the short period of a half-century. Cabanis addressed the physical in terms of the "sensitivity" of the uterus, and he was most concerned with asserting the moral role of government as a counterweight to the excesses of popular sovereignty that he had witnessed during the Terror. Villermé was preoccupied with the incidence of disease among working women, which he invoked to envision a role for science in the government address of social inequality and social conflict in industrial society. Both, however, saw the practice of scientific rationality and the moral function of government as symbiotic, and both intended that relationship to be realized through the investigation and regulation of women's domestic roles and responsibilities.

By defining the immoral practices of industrial workers, and especially women, as contagious, Villermé followed the lines of Cabanis's vision of the relationship between science and the moral functions of government.[41] But his treatise also contained incomplete explanations, both of disease and poverty, that in the end betrayed his inability or unwillingness to dissociate morality from the rational capacities of individuals that had been so integral to Cabanis's understanding of hygiene. Villermé's explanation of the relationship between men's work and disease was ambiguous. At best, he could not completely avoid the indictment of industrial capitalist practices as the cause of disease among male factory workers, but rather mediated their influence through the moral problems provided by women's neglect of their domestic duties. At worst, his attempts at explanation broke down; he invoked the problem of disease among the industrial poor without assigning to it either a moral or an economic cause. Thus, in attempting to explain the cause of high infant mortality among working-class families in Mulhouse, he concluded: "I don't know."[42] And, in what has become the most oft-quoted passage from his treatise, Villermé appealed to his readers' fear and imagination, and not their reason, as a way of convincing them of the need for governmental social policy:

> I would rather add nothing to this description of hideous things which reveal, at a glance, the profound misery of these unhappy inhabitants; but I must say that in several of the beds of which I have just spoken I have seen individuals of both sexes and of very different ages lying together, most of them without nightshirts and repulsively dirty. Father, mother, the aged, children, adults, all pressed, stacked together. I stop. The reader will complete the picture, but I warn him that if he wishes it to be accurate, his imagination must not recoil before any of the disgusting mysteries performed on these impure beds, in the midst of obscurity and drunkenness.[43]

These explanatory ambiguities expressed Villermé's reluctance to forgo a commitment to moral individualism that would make industrialists and workers, and not the state, responsible for the regulation of social problems. If recognition of the "deadly influence of families" as the cause both of disease and poverty enabled government to assume a moral regulation of poverty without contradicting its commitment to industrial liberty, did not industrial liberty create that "influence" by attracting women and children into the factories as cheap labor for the sake of maximizing the manufacturer's profits? Shouldn't the rational capacity that made the industrialist free to pursue profits also instill in him compassion about the plight of children workers? And even where Villermé advocated state intervention in the working-class home to remove the conditions of contagious immorality, he envisioned that such an intervention ideally would end up restoring to workers their capacity for moral self-regulation. It is not surprising then that, in the protracted debates over the passing of a child labor law, French legislators invoked Villermé's work both to support and reject the possibility of state intervention in the problem of poverty.[44]

The difficulty that Villermé faced in defining the relationship between science and government regulation of morality, serious as it was, ended up serving as a catalyst rather than an obstacle to further discussions about the problem of poverty. Indeed, it was the lapses and contradictions in the terms, methods, and conclusions of his otherwise brilliant analysis that encouraged subsequent investigators, with different understandings of industrial and urban social problems, to adopt contagion as a way of conceiving the possibilities of government regulation. Contagion, and the problem of disease more generally, were prominent in two works "compensated" in 1840 by academy-sponsored competitions on the topic of poverty. The first, written by the prefectoral bureau chief Honoré Frégier, will be considered in the next chapter. The second compensated submission, entitled *De la misère des classes laborieuses en Angleterre et en France*, was the work of Eugène Buret, a publicist and disciple of the economist Léonard-Simonde de Sismondi.

### Buret

Buret took as the basis for his investigation of poverty the criticism of classical political economy put forward by economists who had matured in the context of industrial social problems between 1820 and 1840. That criticism aimed at exposing as abstract (and thus untenable) what political economy had posited as a fundamental natural law: the pursuit of individual economic interest and the creation of wealth as a source of social order. The advent of industrial capitalism, these critics argued, did not prove the identity between the production of wealth and social happiness or social order. Rather, it revealed and created unequal, antagonistic social groups: wealthy industrialists and suffering workers. This new generation of economists argued that the production of wealth could create human happiness and social order only if government recognized and addressed the real conditions of social suffering of workers who had been dispossessed of the goods they helped to produce.[45]

It was Buret's familiarity with the theories and critical reevaluations of political economy that explains, in part, the many and prominent references to contagion (and disease more generally) in his investigation of the causes of poverty. Beginning with Adam Smith, the couplet "health and wealth" had figured prominently in the discourse of political economy to signify the human progress that would be realized by embracing the free play of individual interest and by dismantling state mercantilist policies in favor of free markets.[46] For those (like Buret) who were critical of the abstractions of political economy, replacing the couplet of "health and wealth" with "disease and wealth" was an attempt to disprove this prediction of progress by conjuring up the suffering produced by industrial capitalism. The prominent position of disease in economic theory also helps clarify Buret's relationship to Villermé's work; he was critical of the hygienist without standing in stark opposition to him or his ideas. Buret depended upon Villermé's prodigious research, which could have been undertaken only by someone with significant official connections. As a student of political economy, he also appreciated how Villermé had used his evidence of disease to articulate government's responsibility to resolve the problem of poverty. He simply disagreed with Villermé's decision to minimize the role of industrial production in his explanation of poverty and his suggestions for its elimination, as well as the larger political vision that informed his explanation. In this regard, Buret presented his own investigation as a necessary corrective to Villermé's incisive but faulty analysis. This mixed attitude was not one-sided: Villermé was the chair of the competition committee that, in the end, recognized the analytical section of Buret's submission while rejecting its policy recommendations.

Buret's analysis, of course, did not allude to the highly contested (because politicized) understandings of the relationship between disease and poverty—about how poverty might cause disease or what the incidence of disease in industrial society might reveal about the nature of poverty. Rather, he invoked an incontrovertible evidence of disease to lend authority to his own interpretations and policy recommendations. Buret defined poverty as *"misère physique."* Viewed and understood in terms of the palpable signs of disease, poverty could no longer be represented as the transitory phenomenon that political economy claimed it to be. Instead, it revealed a class of suffering and dispossessed workers as a fundamental facet of industrial production. Anticipating the skeptical response of those who would continue to insist that the free pursuit of wealth leads to social harmony and individual happiness, Buret "placed under the eyes of the reader the entire population of scrofulous people, consumptives, deformed and stunted men, exhausted women, and skinny children who are the agents, and we would nearly say the victims, of industry."[47] For Buret, those sickly faces and diseased bodies proved the economic causes of poverty, and he presented cases of contagious disease as a certain measure of the "economic conditions of the inferior classes."[48] He wrote of an English worker with a pregnant wife and child who could find only intermittent work; by the time the worker secured steady employment, he was so sick from undernourishment that he dropped dead at his work bench. But Buret, ever the critic of the scientific pretenses of political economy, did not rely simply on anecdotal evidence; more persuasively, he claimed the ability, like "Ramazzini and his imitators," to fill an entire medical treatise of industrial-related diseases.[49] Buret ended up summoning disease, and the economic causes of poverty it illuminated, to put into question a theory and practice of the production of wealth that, by transforming work into a commodity, had ignored the real and necessary conditions for human happiness—"life, health, morality of many millions of people."[50]

It was these neglected human characteristics of suffering workers that Buret argued should become the focus of government intervention in industrial production. He referred to such an intervention as a "therapeutics" and a "social medicine," thereby demonstrating his appreciation of the connections between scientific explanations of disease and the possibilities of government. By presenting his analysis of and solutions for the problem of poverty as scientific, Buret sought to convince politicians and other academy members to recognize the specific human needs of poor workers that were all too often effaced in political economy's ill-conceived definition of the individual in terms of economic interest. In doing so, however, he did not thereby seek to identify with the workers' movement and its call for social rights. In this regard, Buret's analysis, its economic emphasis notwithstanding, has much more in common with Villermé's moral argument than is immediately evident. Like Villermé, Buret employed the language of disease to define the problem of poverty and its regulation in relation to a larger social interest that transcended the claims of rights-bearing individuals. "Poverty is a question of life or death for societies," he wrote,

> But the vice (produced by poverty) does not remain long at the level of the sick individual, it does not delay in becoming manifest in external acts, dangerous for the whole society, it explodes and menaces. The habit of vice engenders crime. Everything is touched by it . . . the interests of all classes of society are connected by common bonds.[51]

Disease grounded Buret's focus on the human needs of workers, and especially of their economic deprivation, in moral concerns. Through references to the experience of disease among the working poor, he demonstrated how poverty dissolved those social bonds, between husband and wife, parent and child, worker and employer, that were so necessary for the viability of a free social order. It was in defense of this moral interest—of creating solidarity in industrial society—and supported by the evidence of disease, that Buret called for government-sponsored and -implemented economic reform.

Acknowledging their agreement on the moral imperative behind the necessity of government regulation, Buret simply argued that Villermé had mixed up causes and consequences by asserting the moral, instead of economic, causes of poverty. It was this mistake in Buret's view that sometimes led Villermé to pose individual responsibility instead of government intervention as the appropriate solution

to poverty. Even as he pointed out these shortcomings, however, Buret demonstrated the affinity between his work and Villermé's efforts.
Most important in this regard was Buret's reliance on the relationship
between contagion and women workers to define the regulation of
poverty as an endeavor intimately connected to the moral function of
government. In pursuing that connection, he borrowed directly from
Villermé's evidence of prostitution among female industrial workers
in urban centers. "With what frightful contagion prostitution must
spread in the midst of the populations we are studying," Buret wrote.
"[They are] completely disarmed against its attacks, ignorant, de-
voured by a thousand needs, and rendered shameless by the unyield-
ing experience of poverty."[52] Buret invoked the working-class prostitute both to illuminate the moral consequences of poverty and to
demonstrate why individual responsibility was irrelevant to solving
those moral problems. Women constituted the moral force of a free
society, yet they lacked the capacity (Buret's term is *volonté*) and juridical status that defined the autonomous individual. As a result,
women's moral influence depended on the intervention of the state,
an intervention that Buret rendered more compelling by linking
women's unregulated moral practices with the mechanism of contagion. Buret envisioned a state regulation of the economy to guarantee
the necessary "means of subsistence" for families, thereby enabling
women to give up factory work and resume their moral function.
Even Buret's discussion of state moral initiatives not explicitly focused on the working-class family was expressed in gendered and familial terms. He advocated a state-enforced solidarity between
worker and employer that he conceived as a "council of industrial
families" and that would resemble the *conseil des prud'hommes* established by Napoleon I.[53]

The problem of moral contagion perpetrated by the working-class
prostitute nonetheless remained ambiguous in Buret's analysis, and
along with it, the question of how disease might justify a moral role
for the state in industrial society. He argued that "at a certain level of
poverty . . . the young poor girl is necessarily and fatally given up to
prostitution, and it would take more than human will [*volonté humaine*] . . . for her to resist the seductions that lead her into vice."[54]

But was it because the working-class woman did not possess a "*volonté humaine*" to begin with, or because poverty diminished her ability to exercise it, that the state must regulate the "*fléau*" of prostitution? At issue here was the question of whether the state or the individual would be constituted as a moral agent in industrial society. Not surprisingly, and not unlike Villermé, Buret equivocated. Even as he criticized Villermé for mistaking the moral consequences of poverty as its cause, Buret himself posited a reciprocal understanding of the relationship between economic exploitation and immorality that ended up suggesting that workers were responsible for their poverty. Bad economic laws caused poverty, which led many working poor to a life of vice and crime; their immoral ways, in turn, exacerbated their economic and physical suffering. Buret even went so far as to admit that the economic, physical, or moral aspects of poverty could not be measured. Poverty resides in the sphere of subjective experience; it is "morally experienced" and inaccessible to scientific objectification and thus to state regulation. At best, he concluded, scientists could experience poverty by "breathing in for a moment the impure air in which [populations] live or rather in which they become corrupted and die."[55]

It is significant that Buret expressed his confusion over whether morality was an individual or state attribute in terms of the limitations of science. Enlightenment philosophes had envisioned the scientific investigation of social problems, at once grounded in human reason and organized in official academies, as the basis for conceiving state power in a free social order. Buret's faulty analysis of poverty, mired in multiple causes and explanatory obstacles, suggested that the state's assumption of a moral role might be inconsistent with its long-standing commitment to guarantee the conditions for the exercise of individual liberty. In a way similar to Villermé's work, the limitations of Buret's treatise ended up putting into question whether science could inform a practice of government capable of reconciling the tensions between individual liberty and social order as manifested in the problem of poverty. Buret sought to temper (through the regulation of industrial production) the pernicious exaggerations of individual economic interest and right to property so as to realize the human potential—and especially the moral capacity—of workers; in the end, however, he found that he could not do so without (in his view) unfairly restricting the exercise of individual liberty. Instead, Buret could only acknowledge the limitations of the discursive construction of reason that would find in a Science of Man the justifications and techniques for the government regulation of social problems:

> Alas! our intelligence has already shamefully succumbed before the contradictions [of poverty]! The intelligence, so ingenious in discovering the most hidden causes of the phenomena of nature and mind is left behind, blind, mute and even paralyzed, in the presence of poverty which defies it by displaying in broad daylight its causes next to its effects. Our reason lies in the face of the evidence, in order to escape the duties that the truth imposes on it.[56]
>
> The miseries of the human being are as infinite and mysterious as its greatness. The human being is the strangest of all the contrasts, that is, a living contradiction.[57]

For historians, Buret's admission of failure resonates with another and more traumatic event that would occur some eight years later. The Revolution of 1848 was the violent culmination of the confrontation between government and the workers' movement over the question of rights, and an event that the scientific efforts of Villermé and Buret (among others) were intended to avoid. Their lack of success here, however, is not the end of the story. However problematic the contributions of these investigators, they did develop a framework for thinking about and realizing the relationship between science and governmental social regulation that would shape future attempts to resolve the problem of poverty. In the wake of the government repression of the workers' movement in June 1848 and the downfall of the Republic at the hands of Louis Napoleon in 1851, and in the changing contexts of science and politics, hygienists and government officials would pursue a government regulation of poverty that focused, above all, on the working-class dwelling. Contagion would figure prominently in their efforts.

## CHAPTER 2

# The Politics of Insalubriousness

## Introduction: Frégier

Honoré Frégier's *Des classes dangereuses de la population dans les grandes villes et des moyens de les rendre meilleures* (1840) was the third treatise to bring the problem of cholera to bear on the question of governmental social regulation under the July Monarchy. As the title suggests, Frégier's analysis associated poverty with crime. Through that association, Frégier addressed the lack of home life, and thus immorality more generally, as the cause of social problems that afflicted the capital in which he worked and lived. That association also enabled him to define the moral causes of poverty as a danger that made state intervention both legitimate and necessary. "What power governments would find in the moral realm," Frégier argued, "if they only knew how to direct or merely sought to encourage its activity."[1]

In a way similar to the analyses developed by Villermé and Buret, "contagion" was crucial to how Frégier transformed the problem of working-class morality into a matter for government regulation. Construed as a site of contagion, the working-class family illuminated the "hygienic consequences" of the immoral "conditions" of poverty. Both the danger it embodied in its relation to disease and the scientific expertise required to illuminate that danger linked working-class immorality to a greater social interest that would require the intervention of the state.[2] Conceived in terms of a social interest, the regulation of poverty would avoid the controversy over what constituted individual rights, and whether a free, unregulated market or the government guarantee of substantive equality was necessary for the future viability of a free industrial social order. Even as poor individuals and their home life became the object of state intervention, their lives and suffering were considered only as they pertained to a larger social concern often expressed and understood in terms of disease.

Frégier decried the "indecent language" of working-class parents, which spread moral corruption prematurely among children in manufacturing cities.[3] The discovery of sisters who shared the common pursuit of prostitution provided sufficient evidence for him of the moral contagion that operated in these working-class families. Through this focus on prostitution Frégier produced a gendered understanding of poverty that significantly enhanced his ability to advocate a government regulation of working-class immorality without explicitly rejecting the principle of individual liberty. In the matter of social regulation, the state would assume the paternal responsibility, abdicated by drunken fathers and working mothers, of caring for the nation's dependent population.[4] Thus (in what appears as a verbatim lifting of Villermé's remedy to the double problem of disease and immorality) Frégier's proposals for social regulation ended up focusing, above all, on "removing children young and old from the contagious examples of intemperance and immorality that their parents provide."[5]

While much of Frégier's treatise confirmed the images, explanations, and objectives contained in Villermé's and (to a lesser extent) Buret's work, he did make an original contribution to discussions about state social regulation by elaborating specific government initiatives that might result from a scientific approach to social problems. His position as bureau chief at the prefecture of the Seine (the state-appointed official who shared responsibilities for governing Paris with the prefecture of police) ideally suited him for this task. To make clear the need for government regulation of social life, Frégier developed a classification of criminal types in urban society that made the prefectoral servant resemble the pathological anatomist Xavier Bichat. His own acknowledgment of the insufficiencies of his methods and conclusions only suggested the amount of work left to be done by government officials in this endeavor. Frégier praised the superior moral influence that dispensary doctors asserted over prostitutes, especially when compared with the deleterious effects of interventions traditionally undertaken by priests and nuns in this regard. He presented the success of the recent prison reform of solitary confinement in medical terms, demonstrating that prisoners in solitary confinement were less likely to suffer the interrelated dangers of epidemic disease and moral contagion than inmates held in common cells. For Frégier, these examples illuminated the crucial role of medical science in a new and expanded regulatory practice (here, the focus is on the prefectures of the Seine and police). That practice, as Frégier presented it, would supplement the traditional and negative role of government (to repress individual actions that pose a threat to the liberty of others) with prescriptive ones—a *"direction de la volonté"* defined and defended now in terms of a larger social interest.[6]

In 1850, Frégier published a second treatise, *Histoire de l'administration de la police de Paris depuis Philippe-Auguste jusqu'aux États généraux*. Its purpose was to find in France's past a legal foundation for the social regulation he had proposed in his first work. Frégier's reliance on history is evident, above all, in the term "police," the proactive practice of government that (in his view) had achieved its fullest expression under Louis XIV's centralized government and that had been largely discredited by the Revolution's limitation of government in the name of individual liberty.[7] Frégier traced the origin of "policing" to the establishment of the French nation on the île de la Cité during the early Middle Ages. The purpose of policing was to "render the nation sociable." It accomplished this goal, pursued largely through tasks such as street cleaning, sewer construction, street lighting, and fighting epidemic disease, within the parameters of laws and liberty, the defining characteristics of the nascent French nation. "The social order," he argued, "could not exist without laws appropriate to the spirit and customs of the people for whom they are made, nor without a government both determined and empowered

to ensure their execution."[8] "History" also enabled Frégier to understand the vicissitudes of policing as it responded to the growing pains
of the French nation. Here he emphasized the consistent and serious
challenges that political "factions," most notably religious groups and
nobility, posed to the beneficial role of centralized monarchical
power in protecting the liberty of the French nation. These challenges
forced government authority to put aside the loftier, "positive" tasks
of policing for repressive ones. In a comment that made the regulation of disease both illuminate the positive influence of policing and
criticize those who would challenge it, Frégier noted that the government neglect of these duties had facilitated the spread of epidemic
disease throughout the city. No one suffered more from contagion
than those inhabitants who had challenged the social and political
authority of the monarchy; they were rendered susceptible to disease
by "the spirit of faction."[9] It was Louis XIV who, despite a few abuses
of power, had saved the French nation by destroying these factions
and by fostering the development of centralized government. The
benefits of this centralization were evident in the creation of a lieu-
tenant of Paris (the progenitor of the nineteenth-century prefect)
who assumed full control over the administration of Paris, and who
used his authority to construct and clean sewers, build streets, and
organize public transportation.

By ending his study on the eve of the calling of the Estates General, however, Frégier suggested the impossibility of making the history of policing provide a legal justification for governmental social
regulation in post-Revolutionary France. For him, the "social order
that issued forth from this illustrious Assembly was separated from
the past by profound differences. I have not been able to surmount
the boundary between the two. . . ."[10] His silence here is helpful for
understanding the dilemma of nineteenth-century social reformers
who sought to justify a larger government role in addressing the social problems that a free regime both produced and seemed incapable
of resolving. On the one hand, they had found in the "insalubrious
home" the basis for regulating poverty as a social interest without addressing or trespassing on the Revolutionary tenets of political and
economic liberty. And yet, on the other hand, they sought to articu-

late and implement that regulation in a legal framework that since the Revolution had served, above all, to guarantee the possibilities of individualism by limiting government to the defense of formal political rights.

This dilemma defined the first major piece of social legislation in nineteenth-century France: the 1850 Law on Insalubrious Dwellings.[11] The idea for such a law was first proposed by hygienists during the cholera epidemic of 1832. It gained new advocates after the February 1848 Revolution as government investigators and reformers sought a way of addressing the workers' call for state-supported remedies to the problem of poverty.[12] The dilemma became expressed in the conflict between two understandings of the home that were contained in the law—the dangerous site of moral contagion versus the inviolable sphere of individual autonomy—and the practices of prescriptive and limited government that they (respectively) represented. In their writings, government reformers like Villermé and Frégier attempted (not always successfully) to present these two conceptions of the home as necessarily linked; government would remove the conditions that produced moral contagion so that the workers could enjoy the moral benefits of home life necessary for the exercise of individual liberty. But in the legislative arena they conflicted, and that conflict demonstrated the difficulty of conceiving the regulatory mechanism of the law apart from the protection of formal political rights and the practice of limited—negative—government.

### The 1850 Law on Insalubrious Dwellings

The deputy Anatole de Melun drafted the Insalubrious Dwellings Law for legislative consideration in 1849, and his own life hints at the contradictory impulses that informed this early piece of social reform. Melun was a devout Catholic and a prominent proponent of the social catholicism movement that assumed a commanding position in discussions of social reform during the July Monarchy; his brother Armand, who belonged to the Société d'économie charitable, provided Anatole with many of the ideas contained in the law.[13] Anatole de Melun was also a deputy from the industrial department of the

Nord, the primary focus of Villermé's investigations, and he could not have but assimilated the copious anecdotes and compelling conclusions about the dangers of contagion in working-class dwellings provided by this illustrious hygienist.

In discussions of the proposal of law before the legislature in December 1849,[14] Melun indicated how Christianity and hygiene might come together in the task of regulating the insalubrious housing of the poor. Both rejected the well-worn notion that social inequality could be resolved through exhortations to individual responsibility and attempts at self-help. Both looked to social mechanisms beyond the autonomous and self-regulating individual to address the problem of poverty. Here, however, the similarities end and the differences emerge. For Melun, the social power of Catholicism lay in the compassion expressed by the community of the faithful:

> Thank heavens, Christianity has established in our nation deep roots so that each time it is necessary to lend assistance to those who suffer, its favorite children, one is certain to find an echo in the intelligence and the hearts of all.[15]

This reliance on Christian communal compassion as the ideal mechanism of social change could, and did, lead to antistatist ideas in discussions about regulation. But the hygienist's understanding of the dangers posed by the insalubrious dwellings of the poor was nothing if not statist, leading inexorably to the government regulation of the home. Even Melun, whose Christian faith was no doubt sincere, could not help but endorse the statist implications of the hygienist's investigation of the "dangers" contained in the insalubrious dwellings of the poor. "[The] legislator," he argued, "has the duty to eliminate the foyers of corruption which not only consume the homes they infect, but also which most of the time spread around them contagion and death."[16]

However unintentionally, Melun ended up suggesting that Catholic compassion and hygiene prescriptions were equally unsuited to effect the kind of moral transformation that would bring about the elimination of poverty. Catholicism, in the guise of charity, depended too much on a voluntaristic impulse that would remain impotent before escalating social suffering and conflict. Hygiene, organized in Paris under the prefect of police, was too closely associated with the repressive tendencies of government that in the 1830s and 1840s had exacerbated social conflict rather than prevented it. Instead, Melun fell back on an invocation of "the law" as the basis for justifying and enacting the regulation of working-class housing. He did so because he felt it contained enough precedents to validate the diverse and conflicting interpretations that deputies put on the law. Thus, he argued:

> Whether we consider the proposition [of law] as a simple extension of police powers, a legal intervention in the contract between landlord and tenant, or the realization of an idea of morality or public health, we can only recognize in it the rigorous application of the principles embodied in our present legislation.[17]

But when Melun invoked "our present legislation," he focused on one law in particular: the Municipalities Law of 1790. The purpose of this law was to grant municipal autonomy—government by popular sovereignty—to cities over those "police" matters that were of strictly local interest. Here, then, the meaning of Melun's recourse to "the law" becomes clear: He found in it an admirable instrument for reconciling the government's interest in regulating the insalubrious home with other established meanings of the home as the basis of private property and the instrument of individual (moral) autonomy.

The provisions of the law reflected the attempt to achieve such a reconciliation. Municipalities were not obligated to implement the law; it could be left to the decision of popularly elected municipal councils. The regulation pertained only to rented dwellings and only to "inherent" causes of insalubriousness that resulted from the landlord's lack of upkeep of the apartment and its *dépendances* (stairways, corridors, courtyards), and not from the personal negligence of the tenant. The purpose here was to empower an intervention that might eliminate the most egregious social inequalities between landlord and tenant so as to "stimulate" in both parties (and in a way similar to the intended effect of this law upon elected municipal officials) "the zeal of people who take responsibility for their own interests."[18] To avoid any "arbitrary" or "inquisitorial" government intervention into the home that might hamper the stimulation of this individualistic zeal, the implementation of the law did not rely on the departmental public health councils that had been created in 1848 under the auspices of state-appointed prefects and thus associated with the repressive potential of state power.[19] Local commissions could not initiate investigations of suspected health violations by landlords, but could act only upon receipt of a tenant complaint. Commissions that concurred in the validity of the tenant complaint had no enforcement power (exécution d'office), relying instead on the authority of the municipal council for enforcement (which, in respect to this law, was limited to an anemic fine ranging from fifteen to one hundred francs).

While the law passed easily, it had its share of critics. No one was more forceful in criticizing the proposed legislation than Théophile Roussel, a doctor and future member of the Academies of Medicine and of Moral and Political Sciences who as a senator would also assume a formative role in Third Republic child legislation.[20] In legislative discussions of the proposed law, Roussel masterfully exposed the contradiction of invoking the values and institutions associated with individual liberty and popular sovereignty to justify and implement the government regulation of social problems posed in terms of public health. Focusing exclusively on the public health arguments that Melun himself had offered, Roussel argued that the "danger," at once biological and moral, embodied in the insalubrious dwelling indicated a social interest that could not be administered by individual initiative or a popularly elected council. Roussel showed Melun's attempt to fit such a social regulation into a legal framework informed by individual liberty to be both contradictory and dangerous. He noted the absurdity of enacting a law whose implementation would nonetheless remain optional. And he criticized a law that claimed to regulate the hygienic consequences of immoral practices while at the same time excluding the recently created departmental (prefectoral) public health councils. After all, he argued, hygienists had originally formulated the idea of how physical "conditions" influence the moral functions of the home, and they alone remained competent to explain and regulate the causes of insalubrious dwellings.[21]

Melun responded to Roussel's criticism in the same way he had dealt earlier in the discussion with his own listing of incommensurate principles that might justify such a law: He invoked the 1790 Law on Municipalities. But in the end, even this law would not allow him to gloss over the conflict between the advocacy of a government regulation of social problems centered on the working-class dwelling and a continued commitment to individual liberty. For what made this law such a potent symbol and instrument of government in a free social order was that it limited government intervention to the repression of those acts (occurring in nature or committed by individuals) that interfered with the enjoyment of liberty. Accordingly, the law limited government regulation of the home to repressing intermittent dangers—such as flowerpots falling from windowsills or cases of epidemic disease.[22] Such a law could neither justify an ongoing and regularized government intervention in the moral life of the poor nor produce the positive "moral effect" that Melun himself regarded as constituting the innovation of the Law on Insalubrious Dwellings. Far from achieving the heroic feat of constituting a new realm of social regulation, the Melun Law (as it became known) ended up confirming a repressive practice of government intervention it had intended to surpass. That dependence revealed how difficult it would be to create a prescriptive social role for government through a legal structure that associated the possibilities of liberty with limited, "negative" government. The failure of the 1850 law to articulate a new and effective government regulation of social problems was most starkly manifested in Paris. There, the implementation of the law by the prefect of the Seine became the basis for a conflict with the prefect of police, whose own jurisdiction over the regulation of insalubriousness exemplified the continued relevance of "negative" modes of government aimed at repressing threats to individual liberty.

## The Conflict of Attributions

The role ascribed to the prefect of the Seine in implementing the Law on Insalubrious Dwellings in Paris reflected the exceptional status of the capital among French cities. Such an exceptional status was already recognized in the 1790 Law on Municipalities, which did not include provisions for governing Paris. As the capital of a centralized nation, Paris was regarded by Revolutionary politicians as possessing a unique proclivity for social and political disorder, and they thus concluded that its rule could not be left to an elected council or mayor. Instead, Paris would be governed according to the Law of 12 Messidor An VIII (June 30, 1800), which created two state-appointed prefects—the prefect of the Seine and the prefect of police.[23] The prefect of the Seine, who assumed what approximated a mayoral role in consultation with a municipal council (elected by a limited franchise for the first time in 1834), was responsible largely for public works projects such as the widening of streets and the mainte-nance of public buildings and monuments. Until the early 1850s, however, such aspirations and plans were limited by a bourgeois ethos that affirmed restrained government and fiscal austerity.[24] It was the prefect of police who predominated in the government of Paris. He was in charge of those repressive municipal police functions that included making the streets safe for residents (the regulation of epidemic disease was included under this rubric), political policing (such as the repression of the printing and circulation of "seditious" materials), and judicial policing (the investigation and punishment of crimes)—all attributes that aimed at securing individual liberty against the dangers of urban social life and that were also crucial to the security of the state.[25]

The 1850 Law on Insalubrious Dwellings coincided with, and sig-nificantly contributed to, a transformation in the governmental attrib-utes of these two prefects and their relationship. That transformation was a central component in Louis Napoleon's ascension from popularly elected president of the Second Republic in 1848 to Napoleon III—emperor of the French nation—in 1852. It also underscores the contin-ued importance of the relationship between disease and the depolitici-zation of the social question in the "government revolution" that char-acterized the move from short-lived Republic to the Second Empire. On the one hand, Napoleon III sought an end to social conflict by de-stroying the political mobilization of rural peasants and urban workers who, in the name of popular sovereignty, had challenged the legitimacy of a Republican government that refused to recognize or guarantee their social rights. He accomplished this largely through his prefectoral servants, who closed down political clubs and nurtured popular support for official government candidates.[26] In a more positive initiative, Napoleon III sought to remove the address of social problems from the realm of politics (that is, claims that the sovereign people made on government in defense of their rights) and instead to make social regulation the basis of an enlarged, and positive, conception of government. Thus, in a classic comment, Louis Napoleon stated: "A government is not a necessary ulcer. . . . It is rather the beneficent motive force of every social organism."[27]

In Paris, this second strategy of government became the motivating force for Georges Haussmann, who assumed the position as prefect of the Seine in 1853 and promptly transformed its operations. Haussmann had already secured his reputation as a devoted Napoleonic servant first as prefect of the Var, and then of the Gironde. In both departments, he ably executed Napoleon's strategy of political repression by closing down clubs and sponsoring official candidates in elections.[28] Once in Paris, however, Haussmann pursued the positive aspect of Napoleon's revolution in government, creating the urban transformations that we now call "modern" Paris: sewers, parks, housing, and a water system. Indeed, Haussmann's "positive" theory of government closely resembled that of Napoleon: "I understand the word 'political' in a different sense than what our parliamentary habits have given it. For me, as you know, the truly political is to govern the country well, to speak moderately and to do a great deal."[29] In realizing this philosophy of government, Haussmann relied largely on the 1850 Insalubrious Dwellings Law, which he interpreted as the defense of a social interest defined by the threat of disease that would require government regulation not only of public space but of private property as well. The 1852 prefectoral decree, which significantly increased the powers of the prefect of the Seine, also invoked public health both to authorize the expropriation of private property that made possible the building of new, wide boulevards in Haussmann's Paris, and to require that landlords furnish their new buildings with hookups to the city's sewer system.[30]

Haussmann employed the concern for salubriousness to extend the "positive" administrative initiatives of the prefecture of the Seine to the detriment of the well-established, and more repressive, governance of the prefect of police. In doing so, he did not conceal his rivalry with the latter. (In his memoirs, Haussmann related how the minister of the interior had recommended to him the post of police prefect, only to be surprised when the provincial servant revealed his own interest in assuming the much less powerful prefecture of the Seine. By the end of his career, Haussmann let it be known, he and not the prefect of police was the emperor's confidant and preferred deputy.)[31] The rivalry between the two prefects reached a climax in 1859 when Haussmann, with the emperor's good graces and the subsequent approval of the courts, removed a number of attributes from the prefect of police that formed the intersection of health concerns and the regulation of public order: lighting; sweeping; washing the streets; removal of mud, snow, ice, and debris; cleaning the sewers and cesspools; and regulating public transportation. Where the prefect of police had undertaken these tasks in the past as part of his responsibility to repress those dangers, whether in public or private space, that might interfere with the maintenance of order so necessary to the enjoyment of individual liberty, Haussmann justified their inclusion under the prefecture of the Seine as part of his effort to make government the provisioner of services, and the administrator of an enlarged public social space and a social interest that at times took precedence over the inviolability of private space and the enjoyment of personal liberty.

Many people—especially those who would emerge at the vanguard of a renascent republicanism in the 1860s—found Haussmann's use of "insalubriousness" to expropriate property and expand the authority of his prefecture as nothing more than a blatant abuse of power that characterized Napoleon's imperial regime.[32] That Haussmann invoked an interest in health to increase and transform prefectoral governance in ways that exceeded the intentions and provisions of the 1850 law is beyond doubt. These suspect acts of government, however, must be understood in the context of an ambiguous law whose professed goal of regulating the insalubrious home as a matter of social interest was curtailed and contradicted by a continued adherence to the principle of the inviolable home as the site of individual autonomy that restricted the role of government in social life. As proof of this, it is interesting to note that while Haussmann took a number of tasks away from the prefect of police in 1859 in the name of promoting salubriousness, he left the crucial task of regulating epidemic disease intact under the authority of his rival.

UNDER THE AUSPICES of a transformed prefecture of the Seine, the Paris Commission on Insalubrious Dwellings achieved a level of activity unmatched by those few other cities that successfully implemented the 1850 law. Between 1851 and 1888, the commission made 76,958 house visits and initiated 42,394 cases: 46 percent of those cases were settled with the cooperation of the landlord; 45 percent were settled only after the intervention of the municipal council; and the remaining 9 percent required recourse to the prefectoral council and the courts.[33] Numbers alone, however, do not sufficiently characterize the efforts of this commission, which focused as well on extending the boundaries of its attributions. Here, once again, the commission both reproduced and illuminated the heady ambitions of its prefectoral boss. Like Haussmann's, the commission's ambitions to extend its power were an attempt to address and surpass the ambiguities of the new law and its mandate to enact a positive government of social life. That address resulted in a conflict between the commission and the prefecture of police over their respective justifications and authority for regulating the insalubrious dwelling.

The first point of conflict crystallized around the distinction between permanent or inherent causes of insalubriousness and those resulting from the personal "enjoyment" of property. As noted above, the Law of 1850 limited commission initiative to the regulation of permanent causes of insalubriousness in apartment dwellings. By doing so, it envisioned an intervention that would remove those conditions of inequality between tenant and landlord that prevented the former from the enjoyment of individual liberty, understood here in terms of the moral influence of domesticity and (eventual) property ownership. Any intervention beyond the address of permanent causes of insalubriousness would violate the principles of private property and the sanctity of the private realm—which, despite its interventionist fervor, the law steadfastly sought to protect—and thus could only be undertaken by the prefect of police when the home posed a threat to social order.

Initially, the commission appeared both to understand and to accept the distinction. Its 1861 report stated:

> If the cause of insalubriousness is not inherent in the property, and it results from the presence of the tenant, the Commission thinks that it has nothing to prescribe to the property owner who in this case cannot be held accountable. It must then inform the appropriate authority of the existence of insalubriousness so that it can remove it. These causes are, moreover, alluded to, for the most part, in the police regulations.[34]

Commission behavior soon contradicted these claims of compliance. As early as the 1852 report, the commission had responded to its own inquiry into the meaning of insalubriousness by stating that it comprised anything that vitiated the air, including both (structural) humidity or the lack of cleanliness produced by tenants. In 1862, the commission broached the "delicate question of law" regarding its authority to consider the absence of water as a permanent cause of insalubriousness. Some years later, Octave Du Mesnil, a prominent hygienist associated with the commission, discounted the need for such legalistic soul-searching on the part of the commission: "It is enough to reread the law of 1850 to see that in no way does it say that the cause of insalubriousness must be *inherent* in the building."[35] In the act of erasing the significance between permanent causes of insalubriousness and those created by personal use of property, commission members ended up assuming the identity and tasks of police. In addition to their responsibility for those permanent causes of insalubriousness that adversely affected the moral capacity of the poor, they began to make scientific pronouncements about the causes of disease and emphasized their role in preventing insalubrious housing from contributing to the spread of epidemics. Thus, in its first report after the cholera epidemic of 1865, the commission instructed the prefect that "when a water supply is lacking, not only the houses that one has addressed [*opéré*] but also the entire neighborhood is infected in a matter of time."[36]

The commission exhibited similar behavior in regard to the question of regulating the *dépendances* of working-class dwellings. These shared spaces—staircases, hallways, and courtyards—figured prominently in official investigations and debates concerning the problem of working-class immorality and its regulation. The attention given to *dépendances* reveals a preoccupation with what was perceived to be the role of the porous boundaries between public and private spaces—and especially those spaces that facilitated contacts between families in working-class apartment buildings—in the "spread" of working-class immorality. In articulating the dangers posed by this porousness, regulators exposed the definitions of public and private as fundamentally political. Rather than serving as a foundation for nineteenth-century conceptions of the relationship between society and government, the boundaries separating public and private space were a malleable product of the changing regulatory imagination of government as it attempted to resolve the problems of poverty and social conflict through a focus on working-class family life.[37]

After a brief discussion, the legislators responsible for drafting the 1850 law agreed that *dépendances* adversely affected the moral capacity of the poor and thus could not be separated from a consideration of those insalubrious conditions inherent in the dwellings proper. But the inclusion of *dépendances* in the 1850 law did not replace the jurisdiction of the prefect of police over these common spaces, which were simultaneously regarded as containing those dangers—such as the conditions for epidemic disease produced by urine in hallways and garbage or stagnant water in courtyards—that the personal abuse of property posed to public order.[38] An 1870 Conseil d'état ruling on a disagreement between the two prefects over the regulation of the left bank communal dwelling "Villa St. Michel" posed the jurisdictional boundaries as relatively easy to ascertain—*dépendances* that were closed off from public access and thus did not pose a threat to public order would fall under the authority of the prefect of the Seine and the Commission on Insalubrious Dwellings. But such a simple statement failed to take into consideration certain ambiguities. After all, a passageway closed off from the public thoroughfare could still pose a threat to public health, and even dangers to public order could have real implications for the moral capacity of the poor. Members of the commission exploited these definitional ambiguities, simultaneously calling for helpful definitions of *dépendances* and interpreting their mandate broadly. Such actions prompted the minister of commerce to complain to the minister of the interior in an 1860 letter that the prefect of the Seine "erroneously considers himself responsible for all questions of insalubriousness."[39]

The commission's trespassing on police territory seems ironic. Legislators regarded the 1850 law as an innovative approach to resolving the problem of poverty in a free society that would supplement the reactive functions of policing with a positive role for government in shaping the morality of the poor. In the end, however, the commission's statements regarding its role in investigating and regulating epidemics reveal how readily it identified with the responsibilities of the prefecture of police and its repressive mode of governing urban life. In understanding this irony, we cannot separate the ambitions of the commission from the problematic definition of its legislative mandate. For what commission members regarded as the arbitrary distinctions between permanent and nonpermanent causes of insalubriousness and the incoherence of the category of *dépendances* resulted from the unwillingness of legislators to reach beyond the Revolutionary conception of the law that limited the role and power of government in a free society—and especially in the home—to the intermittent repression of dangers. In the end, the commission "interpreted" the definitions of "causes" and *dépendances* broadly, precisely because it found in the police concern with the causes of epidemics a more coherent and potent basis for intervention than that provided by the 1850 law.

The superiority of police power in matters regarding insalubrious dwellings resided, above all, in its "*exécution d'office*." The paradox of attempting to legislate a larger and positive intervention in the home without denying the principle of the inviolability of the home resulted in a law with minimal enforcement power. Established police powers, however, were already authorized to enter homes and repress whatever dangers they posed to public order and the interests of liberty. To be sure, the Revolutionary Law on Municipalities (and the Law of 12 Messidor An VIII) placed limits on police powers; in many cases, for example, police could only order the removal of dangers, without specifying the solution for their elimination. In the case of public health, however, these restrictions were largely ignored, and (according to legal scholars), where the rigor of jurisprudence suffered, "general utility" and hygiene greatly benefited.[40] Thus, in that small percentage of cases where landlords refused to comply with findings of insalubriousness, the commission found it necessary to seek the assistance of the prefecture of police in enforcing its findings. At other times, the commission simply usurped police powers, invoking what it believed to be its authority to repress "dangers" contained in the houses under investigation. Such pronouncements were often challenged by landlords, the courts, and legal experts who argued that "dangers" remained outside commission jurisdiction.[41]

The unique and compelling status of issues dealing with public health were, in large part, due to a second characteristic of police power that contributed to the superiority of police intervention over the 1850 law: scientific knowledge. The 1850 law had denied a role to scientific expertise in departmental hygienic councils because they fell under prefectoral auspices and thus were associated with the potentially repressive authority of the state. But soon after the implementation of the 1850 law, the commission realized how the very existence and perception of dangers to be regulated by the police—especially in ill-defined and contested situations like *dépendances* and "permanent" causes—were intimately linked to the police control of the apparatus of hygienic investigation and explanation. In response, the commission began to assert its authority over the regulation of working-class dwellings by invoking scientific knowledge about the causes of insalubriousness. Because such statements were mostly borrowed from reports on epidemic diseases published by the Conseil d'hygiène publique et de salubrité de la Seine (under the jurisdiction of the prefecture of police), they only reinforced the commission's limitations and the superiority of police intervention in questions concerning the regulation of the home.[42]

## *Redefining Policing Under the Third Republic*

It was easy (if simplistic) to explain the ambitions of the commission and the prefect of the Seine as imperial abuses. When, in an attempt to save his regime, Napoleon III began to "liberalize" the Empire in the 1860s, a nascent Republican opposition found an excellent basis for criticizing the regime in the activities of Napoleon's most esteemed servant, Baron Haussmann. Where Haussmann had defended a larger realm of state intervention in the name of protecting a social interest defined by public health, Republican critics like Jules Favre saw government improprieties—most importantly the expropriation of private property and lack of financial accountability—as being incompatible with France's Republican heritage of legality and liberty. Forced to choose between his faithful prefect and the continued existence of the Empire, Napoleon agreed to dismiss Haussmann in 1867. As an acknowledgment that there was more to his government initiatives than Republican critics admitted, Haussmann's esteemed deputy and Director of Streets and Parks, the engineer Adolphe Alphand, remained extremely influential in the prefecture after Haussmann's dismissal. Haussmann's vision for transforming Paris, although scaled back, remained the basis for the prefecture's activities.[43]

Napoleon's defeat in the Franco-Prussian War and the fall of the Empire in 1870 hastened the return of the Republic. But the Parisians' socialist uprising against the provisional and conservative Republic— the Commune of 1871—once again raised questions about the viability of democracy as the basis of a stable social order and what role, if any, the state should assume in creating a moral force that popular sovereignty seemed incapable of sustaining.[44] In Paris, which had long been excluded from the Revolutionary promise of municipal autonomy, these early years of Republican rule nurtured a movement demanding that Paris manage its own interests through a popularly elected council. This campaign intensified after the passage of the 1884 Municipality Law, with renewed demands that Paris not be excluded from the *"droit commun."*[45] This call for self-rule sought to delegitimize the vision of the state-appointed prefect who articulated and made regulations appropriate for governing the social interest. Rather, the prefect's role would be reduced to that of an administrator who implemented what a popularly elected municipal council deemed to be the capital's interest and the best means of protecting it. This role fell to the prefect of the Seine (whose power had already been diminished by the end of the Empire). Now, the movement for municipal autonomy fixed its criticism on the prefect of police; in the highly publicized debates of the Chamber of Deputies, the analysis of the police budget often became entangled with calls for the dissolution of that office.[46]

For the advocates of municipal autonomy, the historical role of police in repressing popular movements seeking the recognition of their political and social rights (the Revolution of 1848 and the Commune represented the two most prominent examples) confirmed the unsuitability of that authority to administer social regulation.[47] In the 1870s and 1880s, the campaign against the prefecture of police came increasingly to focus on its jurisdiction over the regulation of prostitution. A consideration of prostitution is especially relevant here, for its regulation was a pre-eminent manifestation of how a concern for disease informed an enlarged conception of the state as the protector of a social interest in post-Revolutionary France. Not surprisingly, the attack on the regulation of prostitution under the Third Republic prompted the embattled prefect of police to offer a defense of his larger authority over social regulation that took as its reference point the problem of epidemic disease.

It was July Monarchy hygienists who originally conceived and implemented the medical regulation of prostitution under the auspices of the prefect of police. No one was more influential here than Villermé's colleague Parent-Duchâtelet, whose study *De la prostitution dans la ville de Paris considérée sous le rapport de l'hygiène publique, de la morale et de l'administration* achieved "immediate" and worldwide attention.[48] Hygienists saw prostitution as presenting a unique social problem. Because they considered it to be a permanent fixture in urban life, providing a harmless and even salutary social function for those men deprived of conjugal relations, its regulation was not amenable to the established repressive techniques of municipal policing. But hygienists also agreed that prostitution posed a substantial threat to the good bourgeois families whose sons and husbands frequented these *filles de noce* and whose moral and financial integrity was essential to the maintenance of a free social order; thus, the regulation of such a threat could be left neither to individual liberty nor to legislative politics. Hygienists articulated the unique social interest embodied in prostitution and its regulation by linking moral and medical concerns. For them, the prostitute, like the sewer and the insalubrious working-class dwellings that also preoccupied July Monarchy hygienists, embodied the dual threat of moral and physical contagion, spreading syphilis to respectable wives and contaminating young men with a prolonged and dissipated bachelorhood. To contain the threat of contagion, prostitutes, whether associated with the regulated *maison de tolérance* or soliciting independently, were required to register with the prefect of police. And, as part of their registration and ongoing surveillance, they had to submit to humiliating venereal disease checks performed by the prefecture's dispensary.

The regulation achieved at best a mixed success and, according to Alain Corbin, the changing sexual tastes of Parisian men during the Second Empire made both the established forms of prostitution and the means used to regulate them increasingly irrelevant. But it was under the Third Republic that the police regulation of prostitution came under vigorous attack,[49] with legislators and Republican publicists outraged by the arrest of a number of women who were mistaken for prostitutes simply because they walked unaccompanied on Haussmann's *grands boulevards* (some of them subsequently committed suicide during their detention). And they used the arbitrary arrest and repression of these women to attack as contradictory and unacceptable an unlegislated social regulation by police—especially one that focused on protecting and cultivating the moral function of the home—in a republic that sought to establish social order through law and liberty.

Police prefects and bureau chiefs realized that they could find no better justification for the continued existence of their jurisdiction over the regulation of prostitution and other social problems in a Republican regime than the law itself. In printed *mémoires* and *discours* before the Chamber of Deputies and Senate, they invoked the Law of 12 Messidor An VIII. This law, even if it was promulgated by Napoleon I and denied to the capital the Revolutionary promise of municipal autonomy, was nonetheless regarded as possessing the Republican virtue of limiting the exercise of municipal police to the repression of those exceptional circumstances—like epidemic disease—that disturbed public order and thus threatened the exercise of individual liberty. In response to those critics of policing who advocated the destruction of such a repressive *exécution d'office* altogether, these defenders of the prefecture of police only had to remind them of the futile attempts of the Commission on Insalubrious Dwellings to enforce its findings of insalubriousness when landlords proved recalcitrant. In those cases, the commission found it necessary either to request that the prefect of police enforce its findings or usurp police power. But the most vivid example came from the prefect Andrieux, who, at a session of the Chamber of Deputies in 1884, envisaged what would happen to the police regulation of one of the deadliest threats to social order, epidemic disease, if police powers were destroyed:

> I suppose to take an example that happened during my administration, that an epidemic develops in an unhealthy [*malsain*] neighborhood, in the hovels where daylight hardly penetrates; what will the administration do? . . . It will have to undertake exceptional measures, evict the tenants who occupy these buildings, burn their straw mattresses and other contaminated kitchen utensils whose presence would constitute a real danger for public health. In the interior of apartments, it will be necessary to tear off the wallpaper, replaster the walls, all things that the general interest imposes. The prefect of police has the right to do all of this, it can do it by . . . the dispositions of the law of 15 and 24 August [1790]. You transfer to the prefect of the Seine not only the Conseil [d'hygiène publique] but also all that which regards the surveillance of health. Alas, the prefect of the Seine and his agents will, in the event of an epidemic, enter a contaminated house, they will find a citizen at the door to whom one cannot present any law, who will refuse entry and who will exercise his right by refusing so.[50]

Police advocates were equally critical of proposals to transfer the tasks and power of municipal policing to the Paris Municipal Council, while maintaining the authority of police over the repression of political threats. For then there would be two police forces in the city, each with its own enforcement power, which would inevitably lead to professional conflict and social disorder. Once again, one only had to look to the policing pretensions of the commission for confirmation of such a possibility. "Instead of working for the public good," a *mémoire* presented by the prefect of police noted, "these two polices will use their authority to paralyze and discredit each other."[51] More important, such a separation of municipal policing from the state-oriented and explicitly repressive task of political policing would lead to the degeneration of the latter. Without a daily and positive interaction with the population, realized through the mundane activities of garbage collection and hygienic investigation of the local causes of disease, the task of political surveillance would become thoroughly and dangerously repressive. "[Police] can only live through administration," argued the prefect of police.

> It needs permanent relations and points of contact with the population; it needs positive attributes to assist it in governing the *administrés*. . . . A police deprived of administrative attributes would be the most futile [*vain*] of *simulcaires* and the most impotent of institutions. That is a commonplace truth.[52]

In short, the continued existence of the prefect of police, with its established municipal police duties and powers intact, would produce a social regulation best suited to a free Republican regime.

Such a defense of the legality and efficacy of police enforcement powers was not meant to justify the traditional negative conception of government in matters of social regulation, as stated in the Law of 12 Messidor An VIII. Rather, the investment of the *exécution d'office* in the prefect of police made it the appropriate authority for developing an innovative, positive practice of government. Essential to this articulation was an emphasis on the relationship between policing and science, best exemplified by the Conseil d'hygiène publique et de salubrité de la Seine, the institution responsible for investigating and regulating epidemic disease. This scientific institution lacked legal status (Napoleon I had created it by imperial decree in 1802 and it did not obtain legal standing until the Public Health Law of 1902). But, as defenders of the prefect of police demonstrated, if the conseil had no legal status, it nonetheless greatly aided the police in performing its legal functions. Scientific rationality both minimized the opportunities for repressive interventions by police agents and "softened" those interventions deemed necessary for ensuring social order. Science also illuminated the changing conditions of society and thus enabled the police to reassess its regulatory goals and techniques accordingly. Once again, the occasions that required police to enter private dwellings in the task of regulating epidemic disease were invoked to illuminate the salutary and positive influence of science on the policing of social life. Whereas earlier the regulation of the home proved the necessity of maintaining police enforcement powers, it now demonstrated the possibility of restraining these powers (through science) in favor of positive interventions and in a way that could only please Republican defenders of a social order grounded in the rule of law. Thus in the 1884 discussion of the police budget at the Chamber of Deputies, the prefectoral servant Renault praised the prefecture's new method for recording cases of epidemic disease as evidence of how science limited the recourse to repressive interventions:

> Thanks to the initiative that the prefecture of police maintains in matters of hygiene for the needs of health, [it] was able to develop ten or eleven years ago a whole range of services which represent, from the viewpoint of public health and from the viewpoint of the esteem and sympathy which the population holds for it, a considerable progress. . . . The police commissioners, in this instance, do not present themselves as agents of repression, but as agents of protection, assistance, and relief. It is by multiplying this kind of intervention that the function of police will be endowed with a character which softens and tempers the inevitable rigor of its repressive action.[53]

In the end, however, this reliance on science revealed as contradictory the attempt by police to envision its goal of positive government within the boundaries of Republican legalism. For the progressive tendencies of science that ensured a social regulation responsive to the changing material and moral needs of French industrial society also made it impossible to define the objectives and techniques of social regulation in the law. Thus Lépine, the combative prefect of police who at the beginning of the twentieth century defended the prerogatives of his office against criticisms of the illegality of the police regulation of prostitution, argued that "in practice" it was impossible to trace the limits of policing. In Lépine's view, "[The field of policing], according to circumstances, grows and contracts. . . . [I]n police matters, next to the written law there exists an unwritten law."[54]

Something more troubling than bad argumentation or even the inappropriateness of police in the endeavor of positive social regulation was at issue here. Rather, it now appeared unlikely that a positive regulation of social problems could ever be conceived and implemented through Republican legality. The problem was already suggested in the discourse of disease that had shaped this governmental initiative in the 1830s. For disease had framed the question of social inequality as a moral question that could not be adequately addressed by recourse to individual autonomy but that made the possibility of a free social order dependent upon state intervention in the domestic life of the poor. In post-Revolutionary France, however, where the law grounded a conception of a free social order that linked the possibility of individual liberty to the inviolability of the home and limited state intervention, the attempt to legislate a positive social regulation could only lead to contradictory results. This became clear in discussions about prostitution that had initiated the Third Republic's inquiry into the possibilities of governmental social regulation. Thus, Ludovic Trarieux, the president of the Ligue des droits de l'homme who assumed a central role in combating the police regulation of prostitution, ended up arguing in 1895:

> Above all and as a matter of necessity, one must attend to dangers and stop the propagation of wrongs [mal]. If we don't take care of this, contagion will spread with such rapidity that perhaps the entire population would end up being contaminated within the space of less than half a century. The law is here above all for the defense of the social interest and, if the mechanisms of justice cannot support it, it is necessary to look outside those mechanisms. *I would go so far as to say that the law is to a certain extent arbitrary; there is no place for legislation where we can realize rigorous legality only at the detriment of the sanitary condition of the nation.*[55]

The fate of prostitution in modern France realized Trarieux's prediction. Try as they may, critics of the police regulation of prostitution failed to produce a convincing and sound basis for legislating it, and as the Third Republic evolved into a more democratic form of government, legislators became increasingly wary of broaching the issue. The police regulation of prostitution remained intact until the 1960s, when United Nations policy led France to abandon regulation altogether. In their failure to propose a police regulation of social problems within the law, Third Republic defenders of policing nonetheless identified a mode of regulation "outside the established forms of justice" in science itself.

## CHAPTER 3

# The Debate over Contagion, 1860–1902

THE SCIENTIFIC CONTROVERSY over contagion did not disappear once the cholera epidemic of 1832 had subsided. Contagion remained at the forefront of the weekly meetings of one of France's most elite scientific institutions, the Academy of Medicine, addressed as part of a larger discussion of research papers submitted on the topic of the "specificity" of diseases.[1] The topic of what characterizes specific diseases involved the very questions about physiological medicine and the Science of Man that had generated the controversy over contagion in the 1830s: What are the specific physiological laws or properties that produce specific diseases? How do physiological laws go awry to create the morbid expressions that characterize specific diseases? What is the relationship between the operation of physiological laws and the causes of specific diseases, and how might they be reconciled without either denying the autonomous process of human life or embracing the notion of disease as appearing spontaneously (and thus inexplicably) in the body? It is these long-standing questions pertaining to physiological medicine as a Science of Man, and not a conflict between the old, unscientific ideas of spontaneous generation and the emerging science of contagion, that shaped the late-nineteenth-century interest in contagion and that set the stage for the presentation and reception of Pasteur's microbial cause.[2]

Informed as it was by the principles of physiological medicine and the larger Science of Man, these discussions about contagion broached a variety of highly contentious regulatory issues. Of most immediate concern was how a knowledge of the production of specific diseases might support state institutions like the Academy of Medicine in fulfilling their duties to combat and prevent epidemic disease. The concern was not hypothetical: Cholera returned to France in 1849, 1853, 1865, 1873, 1884–85, and 1892. In addition to the immediate and exceptional regulatory issues raised by these epidemics, the Academy of Medicine had a standing committee on epidemics that periodically presented for discussion reports on the incidence of disease in France. The great anatomical pathologist Bouillaud, who assumed a central role in these discussions, aptly expressed how decisively an understanding of contagion and the production of specific diseases would assist the academy in its regulatory responsibilities. Without such knowledge, he argued, "[b]y what right, by virtue of what law, by what principle would we act on glanders differently from that of smallpox, syphilis, rabies?"[3]

A resolution of the interrelated questions of contagion and specificity would not simply shape the government regulation of disease; it also promised in the process to transform the very definition and extent of government itself. Here, explicitly political questions emerged at the center of scientific debates: Who would be responsible for regulating disease (hygienists or engineers, the prefect of police or the prefect of the Seine)? To what extent and by what means could government intervene in social life? Ultimately, as in the past, this complex of scientific and political issues raised by the endeavor of disease explanation and regulation would be articulated and resolved through a single object: the working-class dwelling.

### Contagion Before Pasteur

In the two decades before Pasteur's ascendancy, the question of "specificity" accounts for the problems about disease that academy members chose to address and how they chose to resolve them. In their review of clinical experiments, members expressed concern about the variable symptoms exhibited by animals that were exposed to a common inoculation; they were likewise troubled by the evidence contained in epidemiological reports of a similar variability, as well as a lack of evidence concerning the importation of a contagious cause that might explain the transmission of disease. Members sought to address these problems because they illuminated questions that had preoccupied pathologists, physiologists, and hygienists at least since the cholera epidemic of 1832, questions about how to bring together a role for the body and an external cause in the production of disease: How can a specific disease exhibit such a variety of symptoms? Where is the cause that should explain how a specific disease is produced? In response, members attempted to resolve these tensions by producing complex and tortured etiologies that only ended up making a mockery of the simplicity that was supposed to characterize the operation of specific diseases. In the 1866–67 debate over consumption, Chauffard argued that the inoculation of a tubercular substance produced that disease only by reawakening an already present, and dormant, *tubercule* that subsequently could be spread in a contagious manner to other individuals.[4] During the 1848–49 session, Pellarin argued that cholera began spontaneously as an infectious disease, only later to become a contagious disease transmitted by air and human contact.[5] Bouley affirmed that anthrax was a specific disease with a specific cause, then immediately afterward suggested that the specific cause could change and take the form of a banal influence like "overwork."[6] Guérin encouraged his colleagues to understand the specificity of a pathological cause in terms of the configuration of banal influences that compose it; such a definition of cause, he maintained, would explain the observed variety of morbid symptoms.[7] Guérin also attempted to make sense of the variable expressions and irregular transmission of cholera by positing two forms of the disease, one infectious and spontaneous (*nostras*) and the other contagious and specific (*asiatique*); he adopted a similar "double" etiological formulation to explain the apparent complexity of glanders, while others applied it to typhoid fever by distinguishing between typhoid and "*typhoïdette*."[8]

The fact that these numerous tortured and complex formulations grew out of the tensions inherent in the scientific theory of specificity did not prevent members from defending their pronouncements as the expression of science while criticizing others as mired in what were considered to be the very unscientific philosophical ideas or "language" of morbid spontaneity.[9] Guérin found Magne's attempt to illuminate the general, banal causes in the transmission of glanders as based upon nothing more than "negative demonstrations." He also found Villemin's experimentally verifiable tubercular cause to have been "seen by the eyes of the mind"—that is, "imagined."[10] In the debate over consumption, Barth criticized Guérin's position by adopting his very tactics, stating that the "opponents of contagion" invoke "positive facts" that in reality are only a "vice of logic."[11] Bouillaud said that his colleague Bouley, who at once argued that anthrax is a specific disease and identified overwork as one of its many causes, "is in flagrant contradiction with himself."[12] Where Chauffard, among others, worried about the scientific consequences of some members' tendency to sacrifice clinical observation to experimentation and thus to assert "futile imagination against the brutality of facts," Guéneau de Mussy argued that those members who relied excessively upon observation to elucidate the conditions that accounted for variable patterns of contagion resided in "the domain of subtleties."[13]

It is difficult to reconcile the simplicity of positions signified by the opposition science versus language with the dizzying variety of highly convoluted etiological formulations that aimed at resolving the tensions between a specific, contagious cause and the role of the body in the production of disease. Rather than reflecting two monolithic and contrasting approaches to a knowledge of disease, one aiming at an objectively verifiable cause of disease and the other proffering hypothetical or "literary" understandings of the role of the body, the opposition of science versus language possessed a strategic value: It provided members with a powerful instrument for representing their positions in, and for making sense of, a confusing, contentious, and seemingly irresolvable debate. As the interventions of Guérin (to use only one example) demonstrate, a member who had earned the epithet of a supporter of the language of spontaneity for emphasizing the importance of the body could in turn use that category against members who placed too much emphasis on an imported or inoculated (contagious) agent in the production of disease. But, once having used these categories to defend their understandings of contagion and criticize others, members often felt compelled to amend their statements in a way that conceded ground to their opponents and thus exposed the structural contradictions of specificity that shaped the debate. Bouillaud insisted that a specific cause alone could define a disease as specific, only to subsequently admit the importance of the body in shaping that cause. In the discussion over malignant pustule, Bouillaud concluded: "Concerning the mechanism that generalizes the virus, in this specific case, that is a problem for others. . . . One grants me the virus I asked for, that will satisfy me as the actual agitated cause, and I will reserve for myself until later on the prerogative of studying and discussing the question relating to the mode of production that we have just brought up."[14] Pidoux pointed out (perhaps not without a certain amount of satisfaction) that Villemin himself, upon presenting the *tubercule* as the verifiable cause of consumption, was forced to admit—without explaining— the role of organic individuality in the production of that disease.[15] And Guéneau de Mussy, who found any discussion of the body's role in consumption as inhabiting the "domain of subtleties" and thus as evidence of an inappropriate influence of language in scientific matters, concluded that "the special conditions of terrain and specificity are important, though secondary."[16]

This constant return to the problem of the body in understanding the cause of contagious disease is best understood in relation to the political question of how to imagine the individual as an object of regulation. Indeed, it is this political question that at once endowed the debate over contagion with a structure and explained the difficulties of resolving the tension between the body and cause. That question also forces us to reject the demarcation between contextual factors and scientific knowledge that debate participants often affirmed when they invoked the specter of "language."[17] Even as they distanced themselves from the influence of language, academy members, in ways both implicit and explicit, found in the relevance of the political question of regulation a basis for agreement: How, or whether, they would fashion the body as a factor in the production of contagious disease depended upon how they envisioned the possibilities of regulation. Thus, when Guéneau de Mussy attacked Chauffard's doubts concerning the purported cause of typhoid fever and labeled him a proponent of spontaneity, he did so because "by removing its cause we have the hope of preventing it. The doctrine of M. Chauffard leads to fatalism."[18] But even Pidoux, whose name and work became synonymous with the vilified theory of spontaneous generation, argued that a knowledge of the operations of contagious disease must address the question of cause and in so doing move from a "medicine of the individual" toward "more advanced and more social solutions."[19] Like de Mussy, Pidoux appreciated the potential of a medical understanding of contagion to transform the boundaries of social regulation by providing a new vision of individuals and their relations. If he emphasized a larger role for the body than someone like de Mussy was willing to admit, it was both because he worried about the evidence of the variable symptoms of disease and because he recognized that the regulation imposed by an acceptance of contagion would come into conflict with a continuing adherence to the principle of individual liberty.

Participants in these pre-Pasteurian debates did not invent this relationship between science and language by which a knowledge of disease would produce a new understanding of the individual and its regulation. Rather, they brought to the fore the principles of a medical Science of Man as articulated by the early-nineteenth-century Idéologue Cabanis. In doing so, they set the stage for the Pasteurian Revolution, rendering it impossible to define these "pre-Pasteurian" debates about contagion as "prescientific."

## Pasteur

Pasteur's participation in these debates began rather tardily with his 1878 presentation on "the theory of germs."[20] How a young boy reared in a modest family in the Franche-Comté and equipped with a basic formation in chemistry from the elite Parisian École normale supérieur eventually became known as the scientist who revolutionized the theory and regulation of contagious disease, a national hero with an international reputation, has provided more than enough grist for the writer's mill. Pasteur's life and work has been the subject of filial hagiography, medical mythology, collegial evaluation, as well as two recent pathbreaking studies in the history of medical ethics and the sociology of knowledge. The latter two have offered interpretations that place significant emphasis on "context" in understanding Pasteur's work. It is from such a perspective that I want to consider here Pasteur's contribution to the understanding of contagious disease as part of the larger discourse of a Science of Man.[21]

The question of life, and more specifically the attempt to redefine the boundaries between organic and inorganic matter, was a constant and central theme in the complex trajectory of Pasteur's work.[22] This interest in life, so the philosopher François Dagognet has argued, would in turn inevitably bring Pasteur to investigate disease, a phenomenon unique to living things.[23] As a professor of chemistry at the Strasbourg faculty in the 1840s and early 1850s, Pasteur undertook investigations in the field of crystallography, attempting to explain how two crystals of identical chemical (molecular) composition could solidify, or arrange themselves, in different ways.[24] Chemists before him, including the renowned Jean-Baptiste Dumas, had explained this simultaneous identity and difference as the product of a chemical process of molecular breakdown. For Pasteur, the structural difference indicated a more profound transformation that, in his view, could follow only from the intervention of a living agent. Pasteur brought a similar approach to bear on the problem of fermentation, which he investigated for more than twenty years after his appointment to the newly created science faculty at Lille in 1854. Whereas earlier chemists had mostly concurred that fermentation was due to a chemical breakdown, Pasteur assumed that the immense difference in chemical composition between the fermenting material and the resulting fermentation indicated a more complex "vital" process. Pasteur explained fermentation as the product of the nutritional process of a microorganism, and he accounted for differences in fermentation in terms of both the specific microorganism involved and the composition of the medium where the microorganism satisfied its nutritional requirements. In his later work on alcoholic fermentation, Pasteur would elaborate the laboratory techniques that enabled him to demonstrate the physiological properties of fermentation through the isolation and cultivation of specific microorganisms in controlled media.

In the eighteenth and nineteenth centuries, fermentation was considered a form of disease.[25] By linking fermentation to the nutritional requirements of a living organism, Pasteur was both engaging in, and transforming the established understanding of, the relationship between life and disease. In his understanding of fermentation, Pasteur did not present disease (as early proponents of physiological medicine did) as a form of human life gone awry, but as a form of life in itself.[26] In doing so, he extracted the operations of the cause of disease from what those previous scientists had come to regard as the obfuscating influence of the human body and thus made possible the principle of "morbid exteriority."[27] Pasteur's demonstration of a cause of disease that could be isolated, studied, and acted upon did not render irrelevant a role for the human body in the production of disease. For if virulence was an expression of the nutritional requirements of the microorganism, then its life could be known and regulated through attention to the nutritional media, including (among others) the human body. In his later pathbreaking work on the variation of virulence, Pasteur attempted to go beyond a consideration of the human body as an inert media by demonstrating how, in a process of adaptation, human life could both shape and be shaped by the microorganism's virulent (nutritional) properties.

What Pasteur had suggested so schematically for the future of pathology in his study of fermentation, he pursued rigorously in his study of anthrax. Undertaken in the late 1870s and 1880s, Pasteur's investigation of anthrax constituted (along with rabies) his most important contribution to pathology, and it often served as the reference point in subsequent debates over his microbial theory of disease.[28] Even before Pasteur broached the problem of anthrax, this disease, which was a "major killer of sheep," had received considerable scientific attention.[29] In the 1850s Pierre Rayer and Casimir Davaine had found rod-bacteria in the blood of animals that had died of anthrax. Influenced by Pasteur's work on fermentation, they attempted to demonstrate the rod-bacterium as the cause of the disease by inoculating healthy cattle with the infected blood. While these inoculations proved largely successful in revealing the "coincidence" of bacteria and illness, certain troubling questions remained that hampered their attempt to define the bacterium as the cause of anthrax. Why couldn't the organism be found in the carcasses of animals that had died from the disease? And why did the disease appear sporadically, at certain times and in certain places, without any trace of transmission from an infected or sick animal?

Pasteur brought his laboratory technique to the resolution of these problems. He began by securing a "pure" culture of the microorganism through the practice of successive cultures. The pure culture, inoculated successfully to produce the symptoms of anthrax, provided more reliable evidence for accepting the microorganism as the cause of the disease. It also enabled Pasteur to remove Davaine's and Rayer's obstacles by demonstrating the crucial relationship between the medium and the expression of the microorganism's physiological properties. Thus, Pasteur demonstrated, the blood of an animal infected with anthrax would display the microorganism only if maintained at a certain temperature; some animals, like chickens and frogs, possess a body temperature ill suited for the life of the anthrax microorganism. He also revealed how the competition between the anthrax *bâtonnet* and a banal microbe (*septic vibrio*) for oxygen resulted in the "masking" of the former by the latter. Pasteur's German rival Robert Koch had partially resolved the problem of the erratic timing and geography of anthrax by suggesting that the microorganism could survive indefinitely in a latent form (spore) in the burial ground of diseased cattle, only to reassume its former virulent force under certain conditions. It was Pasteur, however, who took a sample of this spore-infected ground, isolated the anthrax germ from the other microorganisms in the soil, and "cultured" it so as to demonstrate its physiological/morbid capacities.[30]

The laboratory cultivation of the anthrax microorganism in a controlled medium also led to what would be regarded as the crowning achievement of Pasteur's work in pathology: vaccination. In a process that combined hard work and good luck, Pasteur found that the passage of a microorganism through successive animal types led to the attenuation of its virulent (nutritional) properties and that an animal inoculated with such an attenuated microbe could resist subsequent infections normally caused by more virulent forms of that microbe. Pasteur held a public experiment in the commune of Pouilly-Le-Fort (southeast of Paris) on June 2, 1881, in order to demonstrate the efficacy of vaccination based upon the principle of variation of virulence. Twenty-five sheep had been vaccinated with an attenuated strain of the anthrax bacillus on May 5 and May 17; that group, along with another twenty-five previously unvaccinated sheep, were inoculated with a virulent strain on May 31. As Pasteur had predicted, all of the sheep of the first "vaccinated" group were alive by the time of the June 2 demonstrations, while most of the second group had died.[31]

More than any other aspect of his work, the anthrax vaccine exemplifies the relevance of the laboratory culture to resolving the tensions between an external cause and the body in the production of disease, and thus to realizing the regulatory potential of a medical Science of Man. And yet, in the end, the anthrax vaccine, and the principle of variability of virulence that it was meant to prove, exposed the limitations and problems of Pasteurian science. While his experiments offered empirical evidence for the efficacy of the vaccine, Pasteur presented the vaccine as proof of a biological exhaustion theory of immunity—of how the animal environment shapes the possibility of virulence—when in fact he had attenuated the microbe's virulence chemically by treatment with potassium bichromate. For the historian Gerald Geison, Pasteur's "lie" illuminates the ethical transgression of a "real individual scientist who tries to navigate a safe passage between the constraints of empirical evidence on the one hand and personal or social interests on the other."[32] The vaccine, while efficacious, did not support Pasteur's preference for a physiological understanding of virulence and immunity; when a challenger in the guise of the veterinarian Toussaint presented evidence of a chemical theory of vaccination, Pasteur responded by representing his own vaccine falsely as proof of immunization based upon the biological exhaustion theory.

Geison's interpretation, while exciting, does not account for the discursive parameters of the Science of Man that shaped Pasteur's professional and intellectual choices. By understanding Pasteurian science in relation to a larger Science of Man, the problems of the an-̄ thrax vaccine and the principle of variation of virulence emerge as one more failed attempt to secure a cause as the basis for understanding and regulating disease without denying its relationship to the physiological laws of the body. From this vantage point, Pasteur failed on two counts. On the one hand, his attempt to show how the body shaped the multiple virulent expressions of a microbe undercut the microbe's unity as a cause.[33] On the other hand, the laboratory culture, recognized as the hallmark of Pasteur's work, proved inadequate for exploring how the physiological laws of the human body shape microbial virulence. It was these problematic aspects of Pasteur's work that structured the debate over contagion in the Academy of Medicine and beyond during the last quarter of the nineteenth century. As such, they reveal a debate characterized more by an arduous effort to resolve problems in medical science than by a conflict between the proponents of medical knowledge and the supporters of outdated political and philosophical ideas—"language"—about disease. This is not to say that politics did not matter to this debate. For inasmuch as the debate was shaped by the principles summarized by the term Science of Man, questions about the relationship between external cause and the human body in disease continued to be bound up with rethinking "the individual" and its regulation.

IN 1878 PASTEUR, then in the midst of his pathbreaking work on anthrax, delivered his paper on "the theory of germs" before the Academy of Medicine. During those sessions, he neither broached any problems encountered in his work nor acknowledged his place in a larger and ongoing discussion about contagious disease. Instead, Pasteur presented the laboratory cultivation of the microbe as a definitive and complete transformation in the way contagious disease would be understood and regulated:

[To increase] or limit the grandiose power of these infinitely small ones and unmask [*confondre*] the mystery of their action by a simple change of temperature is one of the most compelling facts to show what one can expect from the efforts of science, even in the most hard to get at diseases.[34]

For Pasteur, the laboratory cultivation of the microbial cause of disease invalidated the scientific terrain that had preceded it. In an 1879 paper on anthrax, he argued that "medicine and surgery find themselves today, in my opinion, in a period of transition and crisis. Two currents carry them. The first, which enjoys a number of partisans, is based on a belief in the spontaneity of transmissible diseases. The second is the theory of germs, of a living contagion."[35]

Such assertions did not pass without notice or comment. The pre-eminent anatomical pathologist, Bouillaud, while acknowledging the importance of Pasteur's discovery of the cause "that we had not been able to see," reminded his colleague that (borrowing Pasteur's own term) "old medicine" had first insisted on a contagious cause of disease. "The discoveries of M. Pasteur," Bouillaud argued, "have only been the general confirmation admitted by doctors and surgeons on typhus, rabies, anthrax, glanders." In doing so, Bouillaud continued, those doctors and surgeons drew upon a rigorous conception and practice of science initiated by Bichat's clinical method at the beginning of the century; in short, they approached the investigation of disease according to the principles informing a "Science of Man." Bouillaud concluded, not without a hint of irony, that Pasteur's brief history of medicine had "created imaginary adversaries," thus associating this self-styled revolutionary with the practice of philosophical speculation he claimed to have expelled from the practice of medicine.[36]

It was from the vantage point of a Science of Man, as articulated by Bouillaud, that academy members undertook not a rejection but a critical assessment of the potentials and problems posed by Pasteur's theory of germs. And problems there were. Pasteur supported his theory of germs with evidence of germs cultivated for chicken cholera, septicaemia, and anthrax—not the kind of diseases that would win over an academy preoccupied with recurring cholera epidemics and the ever-present dangers of typhoid fever and tuberculosis.[37] It was Pasteur's German rivals who led the way in microbiological classification and morphology, identifying the agents of typhoid fever (Eberth and Gaffky 1880, 1884), cholera (Koch 1884), tuberculosis (Koch 1882), and diphtheria (Klebs and Loeffler 1883–84).[38] But even these discoveries drew skeptical evaluations from academy members who concluded that the variability of their manifestations rendered it difficult to consider them unified, specific causes of disease.[39] The inability to produce typhoid fever by means of an inoculation containing the Eberth bacillus, coupled with the variable manifestations of this microbe, led to an alternative and highly popular theory that this supposedly specific cause of typhoid fever was nothing more than a transformed version of the banal e-coli germ.[40]

If, as Pasteur claimed and academy members wanted to believe, proof of the value of a microbial cause was to be found in its application to the regulation of disease, then the formulation of vaccines by the beginning of the twentieth century for only two diseases—rabies and diphtheria—did not bode well for the effectiveness or popularity of Pasteur's theory of germs. Often, doctors and public health officials could not find the microbe in examinations of patients stricken with contagious diseases; and when they could, the discovery came too late to help the patient or to prevent him or her from transmitting the disease to others. To aid in the early detection of disease that laboratory techniques could not provide, new clinical devices were devised, such as Dr. Créhan's *mesure spirométrique*, an auscultation-like device that would enable the doctor to listen for hidden tuberculosis lesions in the chest.[41] Even Pasteur admitted that the best way to diagnose cases of anthrax in the animal skin industries was for workers to look out for the "smallest effluvia" on their skin.[42]

The variable patterns of disease provided another basis for questioning Pasteur's theory of germs. In reviewing twenty years of experience with diphtheria, the magisterial hygiene textbook edited by Léon Bernard and Robert Debré commented upon the irregularity of that disease, "touching one while sparing another, leaping easily from one house to another far away . . . as if it cared little about the law of contacts and rendering it impossible sometimes to seize the link existing between the different cases."[43] If the microbe caused disease, then how could some members of a family fall ill while others remained healthy? How could irregular transmission be explained? And what would account for the different symptoms exhibited by persons submitted to the same microbial cause? If, Hervieux asked during the academy debate with the presenter of "the theory of germs," Pasteur was correct in stating that the microbe for septicaemia exists everywhere and at all times, why is the number of victims enormous in some places and minuscule in others?[44]

This questioning of Pasteur's theory of germs did not represent a single, monolithic viewpoint, nor did it lead to an easy resolution of the problems posed by the microbial cause. In general, however, those members who participated in this interrogation of Pasteur's work concurred that its limitations concerned Pasteur's inability to take into account the role of organic, or human, individuality in the production of disease. For these members, to bring up individuality was not to reject the microbial cause in favor of morbid spontaneity. Rather they rejected the epistemological premise of Pasteur's microbial cause of disease as an entity that existed independent of the body and that could be known through the practice of laboratory cultures. The conception and practice of morbid exteriority, the prominent hygienist Léon Colin argued, could only end up—despite Pasteur's attempt at explaining "variation of virulence"—considering the human organism as a *"milieu inerte."*[45] In place of Pasteur's conception of morbid exteriority, Colin and others argued that a recognition of the importance of organic individuality required a social definition of the microbial cause. Such a social perspective constituted neither a perfection nor a rejection of Pasteur's understanding of the microbe; instead, it considered the microbe from an entirely different viewpoint, so that "the most humble investigator knows what Pasteur does not."[46]

The social definition of the microbial cause that was articulated in these debates involved three points. First, it recognized how social life could obfuscate the operations of contagion and thus make it difficult to understand the relationship between microbe and body. For Léon Colin, what some took for morbid spontaneity was only apparent, the "result of the artificial circumstances of agglomeration and social relations of different peoples."[47] According to Auguste Ollivier, who served as an active and influential member of the Conseil d'hygiène publique as well as a *professeur agrégé* on the medical school faculty, it was impossible to trace the transmission of disease in cities with four, five, or ten thousand inhabitants.[48] He indicted equally the "coming and going" in the hallways of working-class apartment buildings and modern transportation systems as obfuscating factors. The frequent changes in living quarters undertaken by many Parisian renters made a retrospective analysis of transmission almost impossible.[49] Even the social relations provided by the family, the very bedrock of social life, often rendered it difficult to understand whether tuberculosis was an inherited or acquired (contagious) disease.[50]

But social life did not simply figure into these discussions negatively. These scientists regarded it as providing the necessary conditions for contagion, the constitutive element of the relationship between the microbial cause and the body. Here, an enumeration of the ways in which social life shaped contagion was endless. The tuberculosis expert Joseph Grancher suggested the many opportunities for transmission afforded by Parisian social life:

> Has one reflected upon, before abandoning the doctrine of mediate contagion [*contagion par les choses*]: all of the direct or indirect contacts that inhabitants unknowingly suffer; the distribution of water, of milk, of bread; or the market, the laundry, the streetcars; or the anonymous street relations, the omnibus, etc., which become in times of epidemic so many sources of contagion. How, then, can one be surprised that, in a city like Paris, the inhabitants of distant neighborhoods are hit simultaneously.[51]

In a story related by the hygienist V. Du Claux (and repeated by many others in this debate) to illuminate how social life facilitated transmission, a cab driver informs his passenger, a bourgeois mother accompanied by two children, about the unfortunate plight of a working-class mother and her two croup-stricken children whom he had just delivered to the Hôpital Enfant Jésus. The next day, the two young bourgeois children contracted that disease and died soon after; the mother subsequently went mad and killed herself, leaving behind a third child.[52] But social life also provided a way of understanding how organic individuality shaped transmission. For if, according to participants in these discussions, the quality of lodging and food, the level of exertion at work and leisure, as well as questions of behavior, affected individual organic constitution, then, in their view, these factors were largely determined by social status, and especially whether the sick person was poor or well off.

By addressing simultaneously the transmission of a cause and how individuality might shape it, this social definition of the microbe promised to bridge tensions between cause and body that had hampered previous attempts (including Pasteur's) to explain the operations of contagion. To the extent that "social" inevitably referred to the problem of working-class conditions of existence, it also made explicit how the political question of social regulation might shape the explanation of disease. References to this relationship usually emerged in discussions about the practical disease-fighting measures necessitated by a social definition of the microbe.[53] For members of the academy and other institutions interested in disease regulation, popular methods of treatment and isolation, whether in a hospital or sanatorium, appeared problematic in a way that combined scientific and political concerns.[54] If the conditions of work and home life shaped the body's disposition for disease, what kind of government regulation would be feasible and appropriate here? Could hospitals require patients to remain in a hospital if they were asymptomatic but still contagious? If social relations facilitated transmission, could government prevent patients in hospitals from circulating, limit communication between healthy parents and their stricken children to telephones provided in visiting rooms, or forbid hospital employees from gathering in the cafés that inevitably surrounded hospitals in outlying areas and that were regarded as constituting vectors of contagion (the café Château des Alouettes outside the Aubervilliers Hospital was often invoked as an example)?[55] All of these measures, seriously considered by the academy as well as other medical and public health institutions, were in the end seen as medically ineffective and politically offensive. But the goal here was not simply to provide regulatory measures that were medically effective and respectful of the principle of individual liberty. More important, these discussions suggested, however tentatively, that disease regulation could produce a new principle of social regulation that a recourse to individual liberty did not. Thus, Grancher argued against the German preference for sanatorium treatment for tuberculosis not only because it prevented a working-class father from working for a substantial period of time, but also because, from the viewpoint of the "race," disease regulation should invest in preserving that part of the family that is still healthy.[56]

This social definition of the microbe became associated, above all, with the work of Charles Bouchard and Michel Peter. Bouchard appeared in the debates at the academy and other organizations mainly in the form of citation. As a prominent pathologist associated with the Paris medical faculty, he was either the colleague or mentor—and sometimes both—to many of the most influential participants in these debates over contagion. Here, two published sets of his lectures—*Leçons sur les auto-intoxications dans les maladies* (1885) and *Thérapeutique des maladies infectieuses* (1887–88)—emerged as obligatory points of reference.

Bouchard unequivocally accepted the microbe as the cause that characterizes specific diseases. "We believe," he wrote in his *Thérapeutique*, "that for each pathogenic microbial entity there corresponds a morbid entity; that it is the specificity of the microbe that defines the specificity of the disease."[57] He focused his criticism on Pasteur's theory of morbid exteriority, which from his viewpoint as a clinician failed to account for certain irregularities that characterized the development of contagious diseases. He wondered why lesions associated with a specific contagious disease continued to appear even after any trace of the microbial cause had left the body. He noted that in a sample of autopsies 75 percent contained tubercular lesions that had gone undetected and had healed spontaneously. While the German microbiologist Robert Koch claimed that the virgule bacillus (which he first identified as the cause of cholera) inhabited the intestinal tract, Bouchard could detect it only in the feces of the disease's victims; and even after he had sanitized the intestines of victims, they continued to develop the symptoms associated with cholera. Laboratory animals inoculated with

Koch's vibrio did not produce the disease, and even those courageous researchers inclined to self-experimentation by ingesting the virgule bacillus ended up experiencing only mild vomiting and diarrhea.[58]

Pasteur had explained many of these problems in terms of "variation of virulence," by which the human body can shape, even hinder, the virulent expressions of the microbial cause. Bouchard too focused on virulence, but in a way that surpassed the ambiguities in Pasteur's understanding of it. For where Pasteur had presented virulence simultaneously as a property of the microbe and as dependent upon the body, Bouchard argued that it constituted an expression of the body's nutritional processes gone awry. In this vision of virulence, the microbe serves only as a "primordial cause" that disrupts the physiological laws of nutrition.[59] Without abandoning the notion of cause, Bouchard was thus able to reaffirm the potential of human life to become "illness in force" and not—as Pasteur purportedly did—reduce it to an "inert milieu" where disease develops.[60] By reasserting the principles of a Science of Man in such a fashion, Bouchard could explain away the problems that he had previously encountered. If disease was an expression of a disrupted nutritional function, then symptoms might appear long after the instigating microbe had initiated the process. And the fact that nutritional processes varied from individual to individual would now account for the disparity in symptoms, as well as the capacity of the body in certain cases to correct nutritional processes without producing any morbid symptoms.

For Bouchard, the individualistic character of the nutritional process could be best understood and regulated through its "conditions" or "circumstances":

> In the same individual, at the same age, there exist variations in predisposition according to the state of his or her physical and moral health. The weakening which results from illness increases the predisposition for illness among convalescents; worries and sorrows, insomnia and moral shocks predispose the individual to contract infectious diseases. See what transpires in the hospital for medical students. Overwork and overplay [*excès de plaisir*], all of these things that exhaust young men, prepare them to contract infectious germs; one night without sleep leads to contracting diphtheria.[61]

The importance of these conditions suggested a strategy for combating disease different from microbe hunting or vaccination, the two most often associated with Pasteurian science. Bouchard called for a new alliance with hygiene, aimed at "supporting the forces of the ill person" through attention to the social and moral influences that shape individual nutritional processes.[62]

By focusing on the social conditions that produced both the morbid and healthy manifestations of nutritional processes, Bouchard affirmed the link between a knowledge of disease and the politics of regulation. Indeed, the entirety of Bouchard's work combines rigorous experimental methods and clinical observation with philosophical ruminations on the "individual" that the opposition between "science" and "language" cannot account for. Thus, he wrote in his lectures on "autointoxication" that "the individual is constantly under threat of poisoning; he works, at each and every moment, towards his own destruction."[63] For Bouchard, however, a knowledge of disease did not illuminate the self-destruction undertaken by an individual through the exercise of free will. Rather, Bouchard found in the influence of social conditions upon the individual propensity for disease evidence of how society makes and unmakes man, and he used that evidence to justify a new and more extensive practice of social regulation. Too often, he observed critically, efforts to explain and regulate disease focused upon finding the microbial cause of an epidemic imported from the outside by travelers or ships. Such a strategy, in his opinion, exposed how the explanation and regulation of disease often served to blame social problems upon the "foreigner, the eternal enemy."[64] His definition of contagion as a product of the relationship between social conditions and individual nutritional processes led him instead to indict French society organized around "the unrestricted sale of alcohol, and also poverty, consequence of the new social conditions we have created."[65] In the end, Bouchard's address of the social conditions that produce morbid expressions of nutritional processes posed a political challenge: to rethink the relationship between individual and society and an enlarged role for government in its realization.

In certain respects, a starker contrast to Bouchard could not be found than the life and career of Michel Peter. Whereas Bouchard's participation in these debates took the form of a disembodied corpus of work, Peter contributed to the debates as a highly effective, and thus much maligned, polemicist in the proceedings of the academy.[66] That role earned him a reputation among his colleagues (who booed him frequently) and twentieth-century scholars as the foremost proponent of an outdated and unscientific morbid spontaneity.[67] And yet Peter drew upon Bouchard's work, illuminating in the process the impossibility of situating the participants in these debates in the two dichotomous positions of science and morbid spontaneity. In the end, Peter might have been excessive in his polemical virtuosity, but in doing so he merely exposed and exploited the contradictions of Pasteurian science.

Peter made his most important contributions to the debate over contagion during the sessions devoted to typhoid fever in 1883 and cholera in 1892. His position as a clinician at the Charité Hospital in Paris lent him the authority in this debate by providing him with an interest in and the resources for addressing the problems posed by these diseases. At that institution, he had observed patterns of disease that could not be explained by recourse to the principles and techniques of Pasteur's morbid exteriority. How could cases of typhoid fever, supposedly produced by an identical cause, assume so many different forms? What accounted for the limited contagiousness of cholera? Why had three different germs been identified as the cause of cholera, and why were so many diseases associated with one banal and omnipresent germ, the e-coli? Why did the autopsy of guinea pigs injected with the e-coli consistently reveal the lesions that characterize cholera?

These problems led Peter to undertake an interrogation of the microbe. "Microbe?"

> And to begin with, once the microbe is accepted, is it *cholérique* or *cholériphore*? Generator or carrier? Born in the organism of the first victim or entered from the environment? Autochthonous or heterochthonous? Product or factor? Independent organism or parasite? . . . If one considers as idle and indiscreet these questions which are neither resolved nor close to being so, then where does the microbe reside? in the solids or in

the liquids? in the blood or in the feces? Next, how is it expelled from the body? By this and not by that? or by exhaled air? Now, once expelled from the body, does it fly in the air? Does it become attached to our clothing, our body, live in our hair and under our fingers, thus making us unwitting carriers and evil doers [*portes-microbes inconscientes 'et de malfaiteurs sans le vouloir*]?[68]

The result of such an interrogation, Peter argued, would be to recognize the role of "morbid spontaneity" in the evolution of microbiology.[69] For him, the defining characteristic of that evolution (in an unmistakable acknowledgment of Bouchard) was an understanding of microbial virulence as the product of the human body. The human body could not be considered, as he accused Pasteur of doing, an inert laboratory culture that provides the conditions for the microbe's virulence. Rather, the human body "normally" contains a banal microbe, the e-coli; under certain circumstances, the body endows this microbe with a specific virulence that can produce morbid symptoms and only subsequently serve as an agent of contagion.

Peter, like Bouchard, sought to understand the individualistic expressions of disease through their specific social conditions. This brought him eventually to trespass upon the political terrain of social regulation. If, according to Peter, virulence is a highly individualistic phenomenon, its individuality both follows and defines social types in such a way that

the typhoid fever of this banker who just suffered a financial catastrophe will not be the typhoid fever of the peasant content in his habits and in his thoughts: for the first, typhoid fever with ataxic phenomena; for the second, typhoid fever with congestive or inflammatory phenomena. . . . In a similar manner, can the typhoid fever of a woman of the world worn out by pleasures be that of the working-class girl whose autophagy caused by typhoid fever is preceded by autophagy due to poverty? For the first, an adynamic form with stupor; for the second, the putrid form with hemorrhaging, scabs, etc.[70]

Thus, Peter explained the role of organic individuality in the cholera epidemic of 1884 by noting the preponderance of the "senile, feeble, weak . . . the Hindus of our suburbs and outlying areas." [71] By summarizing the social types of cholera victims as the *"Hindoux de nos faubourgs et de notre banlieue*," he made explicit the link between disease and the politics of regulation. For if (as Bouchard had also argued) Pasteur's conception of morbid exteriority had been used to blame the horrific origins of epidemic disease on the different and dangerous peoples of the "East," so Peter intended a focus on organic individuality in disease in part to compel authorities to address the troubling conditions of the working poor in French society.

Peter's analysis of the relationship between disease and social regulation differed from Bouchard's in one poignant way. Peter came from Alsace, and Bouley, a prominent member of the academy, suggested that his ideas were unpatriotic.[72] Such an accusation played on the sentiments of academy members who, in the aftermath of the Franco-Prussian War, were all too willing to interpret Peter's challenge to a national hero like Pasteur and his criticism of French governmental social policy as informed by German sentiments. Peter protested the insinuation, yet not without appreciating how his marginal position empowered him to undertake such a difficult criticism of French science and politics.

### The "New" Hygiene

In focusing on the social conditions of disease, both Bouchard and Peter recognized the limitations of microbiology and pathology in explaining contagion, and they affirmed instead the important role that hygiene would have to assume in this task. Cabanis, in his lectures on the "relationship between the physical and the moral" had envisioned a focus on conditions as central to the development of hygiene as a Science of Man. That focus formed the basis for the development of hygiene around the interconnected realms of disease regulation and social regulation in the 1830s and 1840s. In the end, however, these early efforts of hygiene proved only partially successful, a result best exemplified by the ambiguous position of cause in the investigation of the relationship between disease and social life. For hygienists presented the social conditions of disease not as the cause of cholera but rather as providing approximate empirical correlations between disease and social life that would have to suffice in the face of an elusive cause. This inability to pursue the cause of cholera did not simply reflect the scientific difficulties involved in understanding the laws by which human life could produce morbid manifestations. It also gave expression to a political anxiety about how to reconcile a commitment to individual liberty with the social determinism and advocacy of governmental intervention that were associated with the efforts to explain and regulate disease.

It is this checkered past of hygiene that accounts for how the members of this discipline approached the debates over the relationship between the microbe and contagion in the 1870s and 1880s.[73] Hygienists embraced Pasteur's microbial cause, thereby affirming their commitment to a scientific approach to the problem of disease and distancing themselves from what they considered to be the failures of their earlier and unscientific ("scholastic") past. Apollinaire Bouchardat, whose 1881 *Traité d'hygiène publique et privée* served as the foundation text for a renovated hygiene, argued that "hygiene in order to become scientific [*positive*] must be based upon etiology."[74] At the same time, however, hygienists recognized the limitations of Pasteurian science, arguing that the microbe needed to be reconceived from a social viewpoint and with recourse to the methods of empirical observation. "Return, O my mentors," a student of hygiene exclaimed, "to a more normal appreciation of facts, and when you revise the hygiene regulations, leave for a minute your microscopes which magnify everything . . . even the dangers."[75] In addressing the limitations of Pasteurian science from a social perspective, these hygienists ended up reaffirming the founding principle of their discipline that had defined a knowledge of disease as the basis for reconceiving individual social capacities as an object of government regulation. The eminent hygienist Rochard gave voice to this continuity when he proclaimed that "[t]here is not a social question which is not illuminated by a question of hygiene."[76]

To be sure, such inclusive self-representations of hygiene as both old and new, accepting yet critical of Pasteurian science, are evidence of the sophisticated professional strategies of that discipline. Indeed, hygienists were nothing if not professionally ambitious. In a program that expressed their double identity and aspirations as scientists and government regulators, hygienists sought to "educate" doctors, engineers, architects, and government administrators. To that end, they published encyclopedic tomes, including Bouchardat's *Traité*, Léon Colin's *Traité des maladies épidémiques* (1879), and Jules Arnould's *Nouveau éléments d'hygiène* (1881). They founded a new professional organization, Société de médecine publique, that, in turn, published a new and influential journal, *Revue d'hygiène* (1880). At the same time, hygienists continued their affiliations with such long-standing institutions as the ministerial Comité consultatif d'hygiène publique, the Conseil d'hygiène publique et de salubrité de la Seine, the Academy of Medicine (where they had constituted a "section" since the institution's inception), and the *Annales d'hygiène publique et de médecine légale*, all of which remained crucial forums for discussing the problem of contagious disease and the role of government in its regulation. Ultimately, however, the professional aspirations of hygiene for a role in the interconnected spheres of disease regulation and social regulation cannot be understood as a pre-existing interest that determined the scientific and political choices of its members; rather, such aspirations were articulated only through the arduous efforts to resolve the problems, at once scientific and political, posed by a knowledge of contagion. The contributions of three prominent Third Republic hygienists—Paul Brouardel, Jules Arnould, and Achille Kelsch—suggest that neither these questions nor a professional vision of hygiene were easily resolved.

PAUL BROUARDEL WAS the most renowned hygienist of his generation, the Villermé of the Third Republic. His numerous affiliations at once provided him with enormous influence and reveal the interconnection of scientific, professional, and political issues that shaped hygiene's power at the end of the century. Brouardel was the dean of the Paris medical faculty (where he held a chair in legal medicine), a prolific writer on contagious disease, poisons, and legal issues involving medicine, and an active participant in attempts to reform the medical profession. He served as editor of the *Annales d'hygiène publique*, a member of the Conseil d'hygiène publique and the parliamentary commission to fight tuberculosis, and vice-chair of the ministerial Comité consultatif d'hygiène publique. In this latter capacity, Brouardel would attend legislative sessions to address deputies and senators about the necessity of enacting a public health law to combat contagious disease.[77]

Brouardel also earned a reputation as the most vocal supporter of Pasteur. In a speech he delivered as the outgoing president of the Société de médecine publique, Brouardel sought to convince his colleagues that "Pasteur has substituted an experimental method, which, for those cases where it has been applied, leaves no doubt or uncertainty. M. Pasteur has shown us the reality and shape of some of our hypothetical germs."[78] The measure of Brouardel's support for Pasteur can be found in his willingness to defend, more than other hygienists, pathologists, or clinicians, the tenet of morbid exteriority. His defense of that orthodox Pasteurian position, however, did not prevent him from considering the microbial cause from a social perspective or from insisting upon hygiene's unique competence for undertaking such a consideration. Rather, he found a reconciliation among these competing demands by focusing on the "mode" of microbial transmission in social life. In this endeavor he became the principal proponent of the much-contested water invasion theory of contagious disease.

That theory explained the microbial transmission of contagious disease, and especially cholera and typhoid fever, as a product of water supplies that were infected with feces containing virulent microbes. Brouardel admitted that such a role for water was not apparent; it was this recognition, however, that enabled him to combine a defense of Pasteur with the necessity of a social perspective to be undertaken by hygiene. Aquatic transmission of disease was not apparent, he argued, because social life obscured its operations. The duty of the hygienist, therefore, was to strip away the obfuscating layers of social life so as to reveal microbial transmission as the cause of disease. The institutional organization of the hygiene profession would facilitate this duty, in the process enabling Brouardel to argue for increased prominence and resources for hygiene in the task of regulating disease. On behalf of the Comité consultatif d'hygiène publique, Brouardel often undertook investigations of typhoid fever epidemics in towns and small-to-medium-sized cities throughout France. While the danger of an epidemic in these places might serve as the immediate justification for Brouardel's commission, the task was also motivated by scientific concerns. These smaller agglomerations, because they had "simpler" forms of social life, made it easier to detect and understand the transmission of disease by water supply that was often obfuscated by the "coming and going" of life in modern Paris.[79]

In pursuing this investigatory work, Brouardel proved himself especially adept at utilizing a variety of evidence and techniques. He ordered and evaluated microbiological examinations of local water supplies, which were often completed by his Parisian colleagues associated with the Conseil d'hygiène publique or the medical faculty.[80] He consulted the hospital records of stricken individuals, searching for information about their residence, place of work, and contacts with others that might shed light on the mechanism of transmission. Much of this information he presented on maps, which would palpably demonstrate to the reader how the filiation of cases of disease followed the organization of water supply systems. If successful, these investigations promised to realize multiple goals, linking effective explanation to a more intensive government regulation that could be realized only by enhancing the power and institutional framework of hygienists.

In the end, however, Brouardel found proof of microbial transmission through water only by marginalizing troubling contradictory evidence or explaining it away in what amounted to questionable modes of argumentation. Often times, he could not find the point of importation of a microbe into the water supply, nor could he detect a specific microbe in the supposedly contaminated water.[81] No problem, he countered; the disease-causing microbe had simply left the water supply by the time of the investigation, while (in a response that brought him perilously close to contradicting Pasteur's specificity) the presence of other banal microbes not normally found in healthful drinking supplies suggested that a specifically virulent microbe had once been present also. When local doctors claimed that some individuals who fell ill did not drink from the indicted water supply, Brouardel responded that they probably did and that a closer examination would "bring them under the general rule."[82] Brouardel's inability to produce the specific microbe that would explain the aquatic origins of a typhoid fever epidemic in Le Havre in 1894 led the leading light of that city's active hygiene bureau, Joseph Gibert, to indict instead the role of insalubrious housing. The Parisian expert, however, remained unconvinced, embracing the fact that all of the victims drank from the same water source as proof of his aquatic theory.[83]

Brouardel could have addressed the difficulties he encountered in identifying the importation or transmission of a microbial cause through another explanation of contagion that focused on the role of the body. But his official investigations avoided this alternative. He dealt with the variable symptoms encountered in typhoid fever by calling for the establishment of a second nosological category, "*typhoïdette*."[84] In doing so, he did not so much deny the importance of human receptivity in the production of disease, as judge it irrelevant or of secondary importance for the issue at hand. In a paper on the transmission of typhoid fever that he delivered before the 1887 International Congress of Hygiene and Demography, he concluded that "this is not the place to investigate why members of a group submitted to the same morbid influence present such different forms of the same illness. . . . All of these questions carry us too far away."[85] And when Gibert focused on insalubrious housing to pose the hygienic habits of the poor as a crucial factor in the Le Havre typhoid fever epidemic, Brouardel responded that its role "comes chronologically in second place. It is first necessary that the germ be imported, that it land in these crowded apartments and thrive there. If the germ is not imported, crowding will not create the disease."[86]

In other situations where he did not officially represent the state, however, Brouardel offered an explanation of disease that focused on the role of the body. Thus, in a speech that he delivered at the Sorbonne, for the Association for the Progress of the Sciences, and that was attended by bourgeois "ladies," Brouardel talked about the problem of the body that serves as a receptacle and disseminator of germs. Putting his aquatic theory to the side, he informed members of his audience that "the sick person is the most active agent of propagation."[87] At the same time, he attempted to minimize the anxiety that the specter of the omnipresent contagious individual might instill in his audience members by assuring them that seven or eight of every ten cases of transmission (his reference is to cholera) remained "sterile." Here, he argued, human physiology, and the social conditions that shape it, were crucial to understanding the mechanism of contagion. As an example, he proposed that an improperly functioning kidney could make the individual susceptible to disease, and he argued that alcoholism was largely responsible for kidney malfunction. It was no surprise, then, that alcoholics figured disproportionately in cholera statistics. For Brouardel, the regulatory principles that followed from this focus on the body depended upon the practices of individual responsibility. "Above all, have the most bourgeois habits of sobriety," he concluded, "so that M. Rochard cannot reiterate that if you have been stricken, it's your fault."[88]

In light of the medical conception of specificity that placed emphasis, above all, on simple explanations of disease, Brouardel's "double" etiology is perplexing, if not contradictory. How a champion of Pasteur and of medical science in general could posit such a complex etiology is best understood by attending to the role of professional and social politics in the articulation of scientific explanations of contagion. To this end, it is instructive to note that Brouardel's double etiology reproduced the structure of the regulatory principle of separate spheres. In his role as a state functionary who would bring the explanatory power of science to the task of formulating an official regulation of disease, Brouardel advocated a water-based etiology of contagious disease because it was "easy" in ways both scientific and political. The public regulation of the water supply at once enabled him to eliminate competing etiological factors, provide the hygiene profession with a single goal upon which it could focus its efforts, and allow the state to pursue a program of social regulation that did not reject the long-standing commitment to the Republican principle of limited intervention in social life. By making individuals responsible for questions of receptivity and its social conditions, Brouardel both acknowledged the possible relevance of other etiological factors concerning the body and affirmed the free individual as sovereign in social life, and especially in the family.

In the end, however, Brouardel's politics of social regulation was no less contradictory than his etiological formulation. His attempt to ground the regulation of human receptivity and its social conditions in an enlarged conception of individual responsibility adumbrated in a powerful way the Third Republic's official social vision, soldarism.[89] Hygienic efforts in the home would figure prominently in the solidarist vision that the exercise of individual rights depended upon the individual's prior acceptance of social duties. In the home depicted by Brouardel, however, it is not all individuals who assume the social duties prescribed by hygiene, but the mothers and wives. Brouardel feminized hygiene, defining it as an expression of "*coquetterie*" and "the most beautiful ornament of women."[90] Women's assumption of these duties at once created social order, defined their "destiny" as social beings, and restricted their access to the rights that defined the individual as free and self-regulating. Thus, according to Brouardel, those women who rejected their (hygienic and other social) duties as mothers and wives for work outside the home facilitated the spread of disease in their family that would result in the death of their husband and children, and (eventually) the destruction of social order.[91] By grounding the possibility of hygienic regulation in sexual difference, Brouardel created new possibilities for government to reconcile its commitment to individual liberty and limited state intervention with its ambition to expand regulation. For how could women, deprived of the reason that characterizes individual liberty and autonomy, come to an understanding of their social roles except through the assistance of an expert like Brouardel? He did so, however, only by contradicting the definition of the free individual in terms of the inextricable capacities for rights and duties that served as the basis of his regulatory vision and the larger solidarist ideology.[92]

IN THE 1880s, the hygienist Jules Arnould gained a reputation as Brouardel's *contradicteur*, the foe of an aquatic etiology of typhoid fever. To the task of explaining contagious disease Arnould brought different, although not unimpressive, credentials characteristic of a successful provincial scientist. Whereas Brouardel occupied a chair on the Paris medical faculty, Arnould was associated with the science faculty at Lille. His efforts on behalf of national organizations were limited mainly to his position as a health inspector for the army, which occupied a major barracks at Lille. Like Brouardel, Arnould was a prolific writer, and his hygiene treatise went through multiple editions, including a posthumous one. His significant contributions to the efforts to understand and regulate contagious disease made him a welcomed guest at the Academy of Medicine and Parisian hygiene organizations; but as a provincial scientist, he could attain only "associated" status there.[93]

Arnould's criticism of Brouardel's aquatic theory of contagion and of the principle of morbid exteriority that informed it grew out of a shared conviction that hygiene was best suited to explain and regulate the mechanisms of contagion. Arnould's observation of the incidence of disease in the army and urban, industrial Lille brought him to question Brouardel's theory and to pose instead the problem of the "sporadicity" of typhoid fever. Tracing the movements of stricken soldiers prior to their arrival in the Lille area convinced Arnould that they had no contact with an infected water source. He noted that, in a company of eighty men, only a few became sick with typhoid fever and that their symptoms varied greatly; indeed, some of the milder cases would have been overlooked were it not for Arnould's keen retrospective analysis in search of connections.[94] His profession's proclivity for correlations led him to conclude that recruits issuing from the regions of France with inferior dietary practices usually constituted the most serious among the sporadic cases he observed, and that the rigorous regimen and sometimes unhealthy conditions of army life exacerbated these symptoms.

As a hygienist who lived and worked in Lille, Arnould wondered why a city reputed to have one of the most polluted water supplies nevertheless enjoyed an extremely low rate of typhoid fever. The concentration of cases in the neighborhoods inhabited by Belgians suggested to him a correlation between typhoid fever and the specific characteristics of immigrant life. Thus, he concluded: "I do not doubt that there exists in the outlying communes and in the suburbs of Lille, in the incorporated quarters, working-class people, many of whom are Belgians, more crowding, more negligence, more filth, than in the city proper. But I suspect as well there is more physical exhaustion, less wealth, more poverty and privation, consequently less vitality and abnormal vitality."[95]

In Arnould's view, neither Brouardel's aquatic theory nor Pasteur's morbid exteriority could account for the "universality of cases." "It is not impossible," Arnould admitted regarding the latter, "that the recent discoveries have complicated the situation by increasing uncertainty."[96] Fortified by "natural observation"[97] that was the defining instrument of hygiene, Arnould undertook not a rejection but a critical analysis of the "meaning" of the microbe. "In France, typhoid fever passes as contagious," he concluded impatiently. "One declares this in a perfunctory manner without adequately explaining the meaning thereby attached to the word [contagion]."[98] By thus admitting the question of language as central to understanding the operations of contagion, Arnould did not remove himself from the terrain of science. Anticipating the response of his skeptical colleagues that he supported the worn-out and unscientific idea of morbid spontaneity, Arnould assured them that "this is not for the futile satisfaction of rectifying the meaning of a word and for establishing a doctrinal nuance that I insist on the character and import of sporadic typhoid fever."[99]

Arnould gave many reasons for his opposition to the theory of spontaneous generation, not the least of which was its fatalism that failed to empower hygiene. In his review of a book entitled *Le Choléra n'est ni transmissible ni contagieux*, Arnould thankfully acknowledged that "happily these worn-out ideas are less transmissible than cholera."[100] Instead, science, in the form of the doctrine of specificity, served as the foundation for his inquiry into the meaning of the microbe. He took for granted that typhoid fever was a specific disease with a specific (microbial) cause. But the empirical evidence presented a disease that alternately obeyed the laws of infection and contagion, was sometimes virulent and at other times sterile, and was often traceable to a number of sources including the human body itself. This "complexity" presented scientists like Arnould with a predicament. Either they could accept an explanation of typhoid fever as an infecto-contagious disease characterized by "complex causes" and thus reject the scientific principle of specificity, or affirm typhoid fever as caused by the importation of a microbe and ignore significant conflicting evidence. For Arnould the predicament was hardly academic; as a scientist who advised the army on matters of disease, he was embarrassed about his inability to inform military officers whether sporadic cases really constituted an epidemic, or how to regulate them.

Arnould attempted to surpass these explanatory and regulatory obstacles through "the study of the role of the individual in the production of contagious disease."[101] He argued that the human body normally carried pathogenic microbes and that (in an explicit reference to Bouchard), under certain social conditions, changes in the nutritional processes of the human body either reactivated the virulence of a pathogenic microbe or endowed banal microbes with virulence. This focus on the human body as the carrier of microbes addressed a number of problems. It demystified the phenomenon of sporadicity; what once had appeared to be cases without ties or importation could now be understood as the reactivation of a "carried" germ under certain conditions. Arnould's list of conditions here was impressively large—water, soil, unhygienic living space, fatigue, overwork, diet, temperament, immorality, and "life in common."[102] He could list so many significant social conditions without worrying about the specter of a complex etiology of disease because the body, now defined as the carrier of germs, remained the constant focus of explanation and regulation and thus guaranteed the principle of specificity.

Nor did Arnould worry about appearing to support spontaneous generation. For him, a focus on the body was a necessary precondition for understanding the operations of a microbial cause. He acknowledged that direct (human contact) and indirect (water or air) modes of contagion were possible, although ultimately dependent upon the body's resistance and the social conditions that shape it. Indeed, a focus on the body resolved the etiological predicament so effectively that Arnould was surprised it had not been adopted earlier. "I do not understand for my own part," he confessed, "why one has accepted the transmission of germs which multiply outside the sick individual in excrement or elsewhere and why one has made it so difficult to recognize contagion in the sense of the regeneration of the cause by the human organism."[103]

And yet, despite his incredulity at the lack of support for what seemed to be an ideal etiological formulation, Arnould felt compelled to qualify his own understanding of the role of the body in contagion. In an 1891 article, he admitted its limitations:

> An etiology would be welcome which demonstrates that microbes regularly present in the body's economy and habitually inoffensive, can become infectious and typhogenic when the human nutritive terrain acquires certain properties or the animal cell loses some of its normal properties [of nutrition]. One would understand then at least this individualism of isolated cases, that which one would have formerly considered morbid spontaneity.[104]

In an analysis that explicitly affirmed the links between science and language, Arnould's multiple and conflicting uses of the term "individual" provide a way of understanding the limitations of his etiological inquiry. Where Arnould had once employed the term "individualism" to explain the puzzling patterns of contagion through a focus on the body and its conditions, he ended up employing it to reintroduce the intractable problem of sporadicity and thus express his doubts about the possibility of achieving an explanation and regulation of disease. This transformation in meaning is best explained by addressing a third and explicitly political usage of the term "individual" in Arnould's analysis of the meaning of the microbe.

Arnould did not hesitate to acknowledge the political goals that informed his etiological investigations. He claimed that an understanding of contagion that focused on the human body and its social conditions would distinguish the superiority of modern hygiene among the many "Sciences of Man" devoted to the "evolution of humanity."[105]

In the view of this hygienist, who matured professionally during the external and internal threats posed to French social order by the Franco-Prussian War and the Paris Commune, disciplines like physiology—and even the "old" hygiene of Villermé—had wrongly pursued and identified with a conception of the rational, rights-bearing individual that was at once too abstract and egotistical. Through etiology, a "new" hygiene would redefine the individual as a social being, shaped by "social distinctions" yet united in "solidarity" with the larger "forces" of the nation.[106] In arguing so, Arnould did not want to establish a regulation of disease that would eliminate the possibility of liberty, but rather to find in the problem of contagion and its regulation a basis for establishing a new equilibrium between an egotistical "individual interest" and a compelling "social interest."[107] The social conditions that linked the body to contagion demonstrated that the individual could not be reduced to a free or self-determining being; instead, they provided a way of conceiving and regulating the individual in terms of the destiny of a larger social whole. Such a socialized conception of the individual would increase significantly the presence of government in moral and social questions, an expansion that Arnould supported by denying the adequacy of the traditional division of his discipline into public and private fields. "Such is the hygiene of today," he declared. "It continues to be preoccupied with the well-being of individuals, but only in order to aim at conserving and augmenting the [social] forces."[108]

By advocating that "the sentiment of national solidarity" should arrive "spontaneously and without public powers meddling in it,"[109] however, Arnould demonstrated his failure to establish through the problem of contagion a regulatory power that would reconcile the free play of individual interest with the regulation of the individual in the name of a larger social interest. Far from achieving his goal to frame the possibilities of individual liberty in relation to the larger needs of the nation's "forces," his etiological endeavor resurrected the conflict between liberty and social regulation that often surfaced in discussions about contagion. It was these contradictory political meanings about individualism that contributed to Arnould's hesitant presentation of his otherwise theoretically sophisticated and empirically sound etiology.

ARNOULD'S TENTATIVE ETIOLOGY found its definitive expression in Achille Kelsch's theory of latent germs. Like Arnould, Kelsch was perplexed by the observation of sporadic cases of disease in social life that could not be linked to recognized modes of contagion, whether "mediate" or "immediate." His theory came to focus on a "saprophyte," a banal microbe habitually "hidden in our cavities and our tissues."[110] Under certain conditions that "perturb the acts of life," he argued, the body either activates a microbe's virulence or endows it with a virulence (on this point he reproduces Arnould's ambiguity). Once rendered virulent, the microbe could be transmitted by human contact, air, water supply, or soil. In the final analysis, however, Kelsch maintained that the mechanism of direct contagion was exaggerated and that its success remained dependent upon the receptivity of the body. Consequently, he argued that the variable paths of contagious disease would be most effectively analyzed and regulated not (in an indirect criticism of Brouardel's aquatic theory) "on the banks of the Seine," but "among the principal conditions where one can find situated human collectivities. . . ."[111]

What distinguished Kelsch's theory from other critical analyses of the microbe, especially Arnould's, was the clear and confident use of language by which he questioned long-standing assumptions about contagion and presented controversial new ones. Language assumed a crucial role in how Kelsch formulated the theory of latent germs as a challenge to Pasteur's microbial definition of disease. For if Pasteur (as he stated in one of his early presentations at the Academy of Medicine) judged "rhetoric" as the defining characteristic of outdated and inadequate ideas about disease that would be superseded by explanations grounded in laboratory science, then Kelsch would address the limitations of Pasteurian science by exposing the fallacy of the science versus language opposition. He would accomplish this, above all, by articulating the complex interests—scientific, professional, political—that informed the theory of latency.

Kelsch began his challenge of a Pasteurian understanding of disease by finding in it what Pasteur had studiously denied: a clear association with the realm of language. Such an association could be found in the ideas about germ importation, aquatic transmission, and the Pasteurian principle of morbid exteriority that informed them. In Kelsch's view, these ideas lacked scientific evidence. It was often impossible to trace the origin of an imported germ or to find it in what was assumed to be an infected water supply.[112] If a germ was found there, it was unclear whether the water infected the sick person, or vice versa. The "bacteriologists'" failed attempt to reduce the incidence of typhoid fever through a regulation of the water supply only reinforced these doubts about the possibility of aquatic transmission. Confronted with this lack of evidence, Kelsch could only conclude that the laboratory-based aquatic theory was a "doctrine" based upon "deductions." "There still remain," he asserted, "many obscurities that laboratory science has not succeeded in penetrating, or that it has attempted to substitute with a false clarity, a simplicity of interpretation that does not exist in the reality of things."[113]

Kelsch did not comment on the professional or political interests that might have been served by adopting the ideas of morbid exteriority and aquatic transmission, although the sociologist of science Bruno Latour has suggested what was at stake here.[114] But Kelsch did not hesitate to identify what he saw as the crucial limitation of Pasteurian science in its inability or unwillingness to investigate how the body and its specific social conditions defined microbial virulence. As a social phenomenon, so Kelsch argued, disease could be understood only through recourse to what Pasteurian science had dismissed as old-fashioned ideas and techniques. Autopsies performed by pathological anatomists on apparently healthy soldiers who died from tuberculosis had revealed "old" lesions reactivated under the stressful regimen of military life.[115] And hygiene showed how social conditions caused changes in nutritional processes that either activated or created the virulence of microbes contained in the body. That discipline also suggested how the regulation of those social conditions might eliminate microbial disease. While Pasteur and his supporters had expected the techniques and discoveries of microbiology to remake hygiene on a scientific basis, Kelsch asserted, in a statement suggesting the interplay of scientific and professional issues, that the social perspective of hygiene would render microbiology scientific:

> One was able to believe at the beginning that microbiology would modify the object of epidemiology by substituting the investigation of primary causes for secondary ones: No such thing has happened. It is by acting upon these secondary factors that hygiene has the best chance of fighting against the invisible enemies that surround us.[116]

In what must have been regarded as an especially brash assertion, Kelsch argued that such a modification of microbiology by hygiene would end up offering empirical proof for what was considered by many to be the outdated theory of morbid spontaneity. He did so, not to argue for the superiority of the old over the new, of language over science; rather, he sought to demonstrate that the social perspective of hygiene invalidated the opposition of science versus language altogether. Kelsch presented his theory of latency as bringing together the microbial cause and the body and its social conditions, thereby proving himself at once "faithful" to the "medicine of observation" and a "fervent disciple and practitioner of microbiology." And if he supported morbid spontaneity, it was because the theory fulfilled the criteria of science. "[Morbid] spontaneity," he insisted, "so dear to yesterday's medicine, is not a simple construction of the mind. It constitutes an empirically established fact which one would be gravely mistaken to reject under the pretext that it contradicts microbiological pathology, since the latter accommodates it nicely. Listen to M. Pasteur himself."[117]

Kelsch's theory of latency, which he meant to be polemical and controversial and which was greeted as such, could have only come from someone confident about his expertise and comfortable in his authority. Kelsch possessed the kind of credentials that would attract the attention and earn the respect of his colleagues. He was a member of the academy and the recipient of its coveted Prix Godard (1890), as well as of the Institut's Prix Montyon (1889).[118] He served as an inspector for the army's Service de santé and was appointed a professor at the military college Val-de-grace. But Kelsch did not stake his theory of latency on reputation alone. More persuasively, he provided an impressive amount of evidence that he had gathered in fulfillment of his duties for the army's Comité de santé and as *rapporteur* for the academy's standing Commission on Epidemics. In his efforts on behalf of the army alone, he had observed more than a third of the nation's troops, covering 305 barracks and 133 hospitals; he summarized and analyzed his observations in 549 reports to the ministry of war.[119] In all of these observations, he was "struck" by the number of epidemics that could not be traced to the importation of a germ or the mechanism of mediate or immediate contagion. Instead, these epidemic outbursts followed in the wake of moments of extreme stress and exertion in army life. It was in light of this evidence that Kelsch regretted, in a comment intended at once to expose the gulf between microbial theory and evidence and to play on the national sentiments of academy members, that "the obsession with the bacillus predominates in etiological and prophylactic preoccupations. What good does it do to inflict these ordeals on our military?"[120]

Kelsch's facility for language, his keen sense of the interrelations among scientific, professional, and political issues in the explanation and regulation of disease, was best demonstrated in the prominent position he accorded to the home in his theory of latency. This focus on the home enabled Kelsch to bring together the disparate elements of a social critique of the microbe, initiated by Bouchard, Peter, Arnould, and others, and to improve upon it. The home revealed the social conditions that facilitated the revival of latent germs, while the relations that composed family life made it possible to consider direct and indirect contagion and how they might complement the mechanism of latency. The focus on the home gave hygienists the opportunity to concentrate their efforts on a specific social space. It also addressed what they saw as the inadequacies of earlier regulatory practices. For Kelsch, the identification of the social conditions of the home endorsed a preventive regulation of disease that was both positive and consistent and thus spoke to hygienists' concerns about the ineffectiveness of the repressive and intermittent practices of the past.

Most important, it was through this focus on the home that Kelsch explicitly recognized the interplay of scientific and political interests that had impeded previous attempts to explain contagion. He appreciated the relevance to these discussions of the political meanings of liberty and limited government associated with the home. In recognition of this, he invoked an image, common in regulatory discussions, of a house on fire in order to explain the reluctance of scientists to adopt an explanation and regulation of disease at the expense of individual liberty:

Hygienists seem to me today to be too exclusively oriented toward contagion, importation, direct human transmission. This tendency is natural, for one prefers to blame the fire in his home upon the spark sent by a neighbor rather than upon one's own personal negligence.[121]

Kelsch found in this reluctance yet another example of how, in the interest of protecting the exercise of individual liberty from government intervention, hygienists and other scientists blamed the social causes of disease on various outsiders: immigrants, travelers, and nations. His solution, however, was not to assuage these anxieties by finding in the problem of disease additional "extraordinary" circumstances that would provide the state with exceptional, limited powers to enter the normally inviolable home. Indeed, Kelsch found the issue of "*imprudence personnelle*," of the shame felt by free individuals protective of their private space, irrelevant here. Rather, by defining the home in terms of the ever-present conditions that could at any moment reactivate latent germs, Kelsch sought to make the home serve as the basis for a new and regular positive practice of government social regulation.

Ultimately, Kelsch was not much more successful than Arnould in producing, through the explanation and regulation of disease, a new way of thinking about the relationship between individuals, society, and government. Thus, Kelsch did what Bouchard and Peter (as well as Kelsch himself) had warned against: In the very debate over typhus that served as the context for elaborating his vision of an enhanced practice of government regulation, Kelsch blamed that 1893 epidemic on Algerian immigrants who in his view had served as carriers for the germ (in this respect it is important to note that Kelsch had spent time in Algeria in fulfillment of his army duties). Kelsch used the example of these immigrant carriers to illuminate the mechanism of latency. In doing so he dissociated that etiology from a politics of social regulation centered on the home that had figured so prominently in his theory of latency. Instead, he identified microbe-carrying Algerian "nomads" as posing a permanent danger to French society that could be addressed only by placing them under constant surveillance.

I am inclined to believe that these nomadic groups, which are so dangerous for the population but not for themselves, do not have typhus but carry the cause within them. The vigilance of public hygiene is needed not only in regard to those vagabonds suffering from typhus but also those who are not.[122]

## Tout-à-l'égout

A definitive recognition of the importance of the home for the inter-related tasks of disease and social regulation emerged out of the prolonged intraprofessional debate between engineers and hygienists about dumping human waste in the Paris sewer system—"*tout-à-l'égout.*"[123] This debate, which began in the mid-1870s and which lasted over thirty years, occupying at least six municipal, prefectoral, or ministerial commissions, concerned the problems posed by this most brilliant yet unfinished aspect of Haussmann's rebuilding of Paris. The prefect of the Seine and his assistant, the engineer Eugène Belgrand, had constructed or planned sewer lines for every street in Paris that would empty into three collectors located throughout the city. Plans for the sewer system outlived the political system that had brought Haussmann to power. Yet, by the late 1870s, the plans remained unfinished. Many streets, usually those located in the poorer, older, and dirtier sections of the city, still lacked sewer lines. And if the construction of the sewers was meant to create a cleaner and more healthful capital, then many observers regarded the continued dumping of sewer contents in the Seine as counterproductive. More important, officials had not resolved the problem of what to do with human waste, which collected in cesspools located underneath residential buildings and which was periodically carried off by cesspool workers to the garbage dump of Montfauçon in northern Paris. Officials and residents worried about the possibility of infection resulting from leaks in the pipes that delivered human waste from the toilets to the underground cesspools, as well as careless emptying of cesspools and transport of their contents by cesspool workers. Engineers, who had been responsible for the sewers since their transformation under Haussmann's administration, remained committed to the prefect's original plan and insisted that the system could accommodate the disposal of human waste. An 1874 commission set up by the ministry of public works discussed and accepted the principle of "*tout-à-l'égout.*" The municipal council also accepted the principle in 1876, received seventeen reports either supporting or opposing it, and obtained a definitive report in 1880.

By 1880, however, changed circumstances had rendered problematic this decision to support and extend the scope of Haussmann's sewer project. In the summer of that year, bad odors raised fears among the Parisian populace that the sewers were spreading disease throughout the city, and the minister of agriculture responded by setting up a "smells commission" that included (among others) Pasteur and Brouardel. Their participation was a recognition of the importance of Pasteurian science and the renaissance of hygiene it facilitated. The Société de médecine publique and the International Congress of Hygiene and Demography, both relatively new organizations, heard and published reports on the role of sewers in the transmission of contagious disease, and especially typhoid fever. It was hygienists who reinitiated the campaign against the implementation of *tout-à-l'égout*. Drawing upon their investigations into the fecal origins of typhoid fever, they saw the system as increasing the incidence of disease in many ways. The design of Haussmann's renowned sewer galleries, suffering from inadequate slope and water pressure, enabled materials to stagnate and thus provided a perfect "milieu" for microbial growth and transmission. Dumping sewer contents in the Seine would make that river another milieu for disease, while the plans to carry sewer waste to the communes of Achères and Gennevilliers, where it would serve as fertilizer for agriculture, threatened to export disease to the western suburbs of Paris. (Here, Pasteur's spore theory provided a powerful and frightening example of what could happen.)

In the interests of health, hygienists argued that cesspools should be eliminated and replaced by the creation of a canal, separate from the sewer, that would carry human waste to the ocean. Hygiene arguments proved effective, and the commission decided against *tout-à-l'égout*. Meanwhile, the prefect of the Seine had created a "*commission technique de l'assainissement*" to address the issue of disease. To this end, the prefectoral commission, composed mainly of hygienists and engineers, toured the sewers, observed experiments on the purifying attributes of soil [*épuration*], and visited sewer systems in Brussels, Amsterdam, and London. The commission, with the prominent exception of Brouardel, approved *tout-à-l'égout*, as did the municipal council (again) in 1884.

The problem of *tout-à-l'égout* was far from settled, however. Because the land to be fertilized existed in the public domain, proposals for its use required legislative approval that was given reluctantly and only after much debate and considerable opposition. The costs involved in realizing *tout-à-l'égout* were enormous. To furnish apartment houses with toilets hooked up to the sewer would cost landlords ff2,100 per floor and ff480 a year for water. Georges Bechmann, now the chief engineer for the Seine, estimated the public cost for implementing *tout-à-l'égout* at ff25,000,000, which he and other administrators sought to raise through an obligatory municipal tax on private cesspool pipes (*tuyaux de chute*).[124] The costs created new opposition. A public survey expressed widespread dissatisfaction with the project. A syndicate of landlords organized and effectively expressed opposition, combining property and financial interests with hygienic concerns that only became more pressing with the cholera epidemics of 1884–85 and 1892. Thus, an article published in its journal warned: "Paris poisons Paris and that which surrounds it. If *tout-à-l'égout* is maintained, this will mean the plague for everyone and the ruination of Parisian commerce. Diverse epidemics will exist permanently."[125] Cesspool workers, whose jobs would be eliminated if *tout-à-l'égout* succeeded, also protested. An 1894 prefectoral decree specifying the means for implementing *tout-à-l'égout* was found by the administrative court in 1896 to exceed the prefect's power; a similar excess was found in the prefect's attempt to rely on the 1850 Insalubrious Dwellings Law to realize *tout-à-l'égout*.[126] These legal battles raged on until the eve of World War I. By that time, however, market pressures brought by tenants in search of dwellings with toilets hooked up to the sewer system had motivated landlords to undertake the measures voluntarily. Still, by 1913, 25,821 cesspools existed in the capital.[127]

Historians see in this tardy acceptance of *tout-à-l'égout* the tri-

umph of both the engineers' position and Pasteurian science.[128] Such
an interpretation, however, says either too much or too little. All the
participants in this prolonged debate, and especially the opposing
forces of engineers and hygienists, accepted the microbial cause as the
basis for their arguments about sewers and the spread of disease. Engineers questioned not the microbe but the hygienists' understanding
of it. Durand-Claye, a municipal engineer with the prefecture of the
Seine and a prominent participant in these debates whose award-
winning article on typhoid fever lent him considerable authority in
etiological questions, doubted the scientific validity of the relationship between the sewer and disease put forward by Brouardel and
other hygienists. Viewing their statements as vague and lacking evidence—after all, how could hygienists claim the sewer spread typhoid
fever if its microbial cause had not even been confirmed yet?—
Durand-Claye informed Brouardel and other hygienists, not without
a hint of condescension, that "this is not scientific language."[129]

Marie-Davy, Durand-Claye's colleague and ally in these debates,
likewise portrayed members of his own profession as adhering to scientific standards that hygienists in their turn ignored. In his view, the
statements of engineers were supported by "tangible facts concerning
the causes [of diseases] and are governed by formulations possessing
an algebraic precision," whereas hygienists' conclusions issued from
"absolute and stubborn theoreticians."[130] In order to distinguish their
approach from hygienists' reliance on "negative facts" and argumentation by anomaly or exception, engineers presented "positive facts"
that would indict the "theory" of sewer transmission. They invited
public officials to Gennevilliers, where they prepared meals (to much
acclaim) with vegetables from the fertilized fields. They offered statistics proving that very few sewer workers fell ill with typhoid fever,
and showed that cities like London had adopted *tout-à-l'égout* without a rise in typhoid fever rates. They argued that the odors that occasionally emanated from the sewers did not cause disease, as Pasteur's
recent work had demonstrated.

The origin of germs, engineers concluded, was the individual.
They understood the role of the individual in two distinct ways, both
as a transmitter of germs and as a carrier of latent germs that could be

revived under certain conditions. But the regulation they proposed indicted one space. In the task of combating disease, engineers argued, hygienists should focus their attention not on the sewer, but on the home. "It is the individual who is his own worst enemy and the source that kills him the most often," Marie-Davy argued. "It is necessary to purify the dwelling where our wives and children live."[131]

Hygienists, members of a profession that had regenerated itself around the potentials and problems of Pasteurian science, did not find it difficult to respond to the scientific challenge of engineers. Brouardel confessed that while he would have made a bad engineer, Durand-Claye's "medical erudition is recently acquired."[132] In an 1883 editorial that appeared in the *Revue médical*, Richet posed the same opinion more bluntly: "Engineers know the art of engineering. Do they know what typhoid fever is? Do they know the meaning of the word contagion? . . ."[133] Hygienists admitted that the application of Pasteur's work to the identification and understanding of microbial diseases remained theoretical, hypothetical. But they refused to accept as "scientific" the engineers' conclusion that an unproven mode of transmission posed no risk and should thus be left unregulated. If, according to Brouardel, "a drop of liquid" containing microbes can "sow" one of Pasteur's balloon flasks, then couldn't it, "in time," infect "a million hectoliters contained in a fertile sewer?"[134] For hygienists it would be highly "unscientific," in the current state of knowledge about disease, to expect an absolute law of contagion, as well as to not take seriously the uncertain yet possible risk posed by the sewer. Thus, the hygienist Du Mesnil argued that "we think it would be better to at first proceed as if on this point one possessed certainties and not doubts. . . ."[135] In speeches and letters delivered before the commissions, Pasteur lent his prestige to the hygienists' advocacy of scientific caution. True, Pasteur admitted, a knowledge of contagion was based almost exclusively upon his laboratory investigation of anthrax; here, however, "indisputable facts" existed, and (in a skilled invocation of his authority) he himself would be reluctant to assume responsibility for the implementation of disease regulation that did not address the potential for transmission through the sewer.[136]

In an argument that was especially persuasive because it drew upon their specific expertise concerning social life, hygienists further discounted the criticism of engineers by insisting that many of the uncertainties regarding the relationship between the sewer and disease were only apparent, the result of the obfuscating role of social life that hygienists alone could address. This was especially true for Paris, where "we are at every moment, thanks to our life, in the presence of unknown *foyers* (of disease) at school, in restaurants, in our own homes. . . ."[137] The anonymous and complex character of social life in Paris made it impossible to know, argued Brouardel and other hygienists, whether vegetables grown at Gennevilliers had caused disease because it was impossible to trace the fates of Parisian residents who bought them at Les Halles. "Does one know," asked Brouardel's staunchest supporter, Girard, "who has bought and consumed them?"[138]

What is so fascinating about these debates is how engineers and hygienists, who concurred on so many points, could end up espousing such divergent claims about how to explain and regulate contagion. Everyone accepted Pasteurian science as the framework for considering the problem of disease. Engineers did not deny hygiene's evidence about the fecal origins of typhoid fever, while hygienists agreed (some more than others) that an explanation of disease should take into consideration the role of human receptivity and how it was shaped by the conditions of the home. (As evidence of his support in this regard, Brouardel described the sewer as the direct continuation of the sick intestine.) Yet, in the end, hygienists focused on the sewer, while engineers on the home, and each professional group sought to secure victory for its position by questioning the scientific credentials of the other.

The articulation of these positions is best understood by taking into account the role of professional and political questions in etiology. The Paris sewer system was the great achievement of Haussmann's rebuilding of Paris and the vehicle for the ascendancy of the engineering profession in the Second Empire experiment in social government. It was inconceivable that engineers would entertain the possibility of inadequate slope and circulation in the sewer galleries;

to do so would implicate this engineering marvel in the spread of disease and thus threaten the very basis of that profession's authority in the administration of urban life. Instead, engineers found it safer to emphasize the etiological significance of the home, which, after all, the hygiene profession had pursued vigorously since the 1832 cholera epidemic. This focus on the home, however, had proven to be the stumbling block for hygienists during the Second Empire. Despite the claims of Napoleon III and Haussmann that the regulation of disease would set the stage for a new, and positive, form of social government dissociated from the category of rights, they hesitated to infringe upon the economic and political interests of private property that such an expanded vision of government entailed. In doing so, the Second Empire distanced itself from the hygiene profession, favoring instead engineers and their penchant for monumental public works. This professional frustration, compounded by Napoleon's efforts to strip hygienists with Republican sympathies of their official duties and positions,[139] left hygienists ill-disposed toward their more conservative and influential rivals. By emphasizing the problem of the sewer over the home, hygienists at once avoided difficult questions about private property and challenged the very achievement that would ensure the continued prestige of engineering under the Third Republic.

But the new political circumstances of the Third Republic promised a change in the respective fortunes of the engineering and hygiene professions. On the one hand, the conservatism of engineering, evident in its historical support for imperial regimes and its criticism of radical and socialist supporters of the current government, came to be seen as incompatible with the goals of the fledgling Republic. Critics found evidence of engineering's conservatism, above all, in the discipline's problematic relationship to science. They judged the curriculum of the École polytechnique, the training ground of engineers who sought a career (mainly) in the army and (less so) in civil occupations like urban administration and infrastructure, as too abstract and elitist. The curriculum favored the classics and mathematics, topics that effectively limited matriculation to lycée-trained students. At the same time, the curriculum ignored physiology and chemistry, widely regarded as the pinnacle of French scientific accomplishment and an indispensable instrument in the realization of Republican social reform.[140] Hygienists played on these accusations of engineers' lack of scientific rigor by judging their pronouncements abstract, while engineers tried to demonstrate their scientific credentials by remaking themselves as experts in the field of etiology. Hygienists could assert themselves here because they, and the medical profession more generally, emerged as the leading allies of the Third Republic. Next to the lawyers, they constituted the largest professional representation in the Third Republic legislature. More so than lawyers, however, the medical profession supported the Republican vision for social reform, which its members helped to conceptualize and pursue through knowledge about disease.[141]

If, as this contextualized reading suggests, the debate over *tout-à-l'égout* ended up serving as an important moment in the ascendancy of hygiene, then the profession's progress here would have everything to do with adopting a new perspective on the home. Engineers might have presented their understanding of the relationship between the home and disease as an impossible challenge to their rivals, who had dared to indict the sewer system; but hygienists did not accept it as such. The debate over *tout-à-l'égout* was a crucial moment in the development of hygiene around the question of contagion because it imposed upon its members the necessity of confronting and rethinking the meanings associated with the home. Nothing less was at stake in this endeavor than resolving the relationship between liberty and social regulation that had been at the heart of the debates over contagion since the 1830s.[142]

CHAPTER 4

# The Foyer of Disease

## Introduction: Léon Colin and the "Social Fact"

In his 1885 treatise *Paris: Sa topographie—son hygiène—ses maladies* the noted hygienist Léon Colin found in the ever-present danger of disease the true essence of Haussmann's modern Paris. As he saw it, the construction of new spaces devoted to recreation and leisure—parks, theaters, cafés, and luxurious hotels—had intensified the social life of the capital and thus increased the opportunities for contagious contacts. He also recognized a different kind of *nouveau venu*, the provincial from Limoges or the Var who sought out Paris for employment opportunities created by the booming building trades that accompanied the transformation of the capital. Unacclimated to the rhythms of urban life and often living in dismal conditions, Colin observed, those workers who labored in the creation of Haussmann's Paris also ended up serving as the victims and vectors of contagious disease. He provided evidence of how wealthy tourist and toiling worker alike aggravated the limitations of the new waste-disposal systems that Haussmann's engineering corps had put in place to prevent the incidence of disease; garbage piled up in front of apartment buildings and sewage stagnated in galleries possessing inadequate slope.

For Colin, however, it was the dwelling that unified these sources

of contagious disease and thus best captured the problematic transformations of Haussmann's Paris.[1] Behind the monumental facades
of the new bourgeois apartment buildings in the western sections of
the capital, he discovered small bedrooms deprived of air and sunlight. He explained how the expropriation of slums in the working-
class areas of eastern Paris had reduced the availability of affordable
housing, forcing a growing working population to reside in dilapi-
dated boardinghouses, share the already inadequate and crowded
apartments that had escaped Haussmann's demolitions in the center
of the city, or retreat to the new makeshift *cités* that sprouted over-
night in the recently annexed outlying arrondissements. Colin's conclusion is clear: Where Haussmannization was intended as an experiment in social government to be realized by eradicating the insalubrious dwelling, the persistence of insalubrious dwellings and the
creation of new ones indicted the speculative practices that ended up
dominating that experiment.

For those who might dismiss these problems and continue to
support these speculative practices by noting that most cases of disease were found among the poor and thus reflected the inevitable
inequalities of fortune among individuals in a free social order, Colin
reminded them of the solidarity that linked individuals and neighborhoods in urban life: In the event of an epidemic, there was no
guarantee that an individual, an apartment building, a neighborhood
would be left untouched by disease.[2] To rectify these problems, he
recommended a larger role for the hygiene services associated with
the prefect of police, which in his view would improve upon the well-
publicized weaknesses of the Commission on Insalubrious Dwellings
by providing a more rigorous regulation of urban dwellings.

While Colin's conclusions supported controversial political and
professional interests that included curtailing the enjoyment of private property, the exercise of individual liberty, and the authority of
the prefecture of the Seine, his rigorous observation would have
shaken the joie de vivre of the most ardent pleasure-seeking tourist
and the confidence of the prefectoral administrator. Who could remain unmoved by his detailed description of the *"foyer d'infection"*
constituted by the cité Jeanne d'Arc, "superposition in five stories of a

population numbering more than two thousand inhabitants, in apartments nearly all too small and, except those facing northeast, taking sunlight only from the interior courtyard or the *passage* hardly five meters in length" [3] Who could not appreciate how the concentration of three cases of cholera on the rue Ste. Margueritte during the 1884 epidemic had borne out his prediction about the dangers posed by insalubrious *garnis* in this eastern working-class neighborhood?[4]

Colin did not intend such evidence merely to bring the problem of disease to the attention of Parisian residents and government regulators. His objective was more ambitious and complex: to present the epidemic, and the role of the home in it, as crystallizing a new vision of society informed by a new, more expansive practice of regulation.[5] In doing so, Colin conceived the epidemic as a social fact that informed so many other Third Republic social initiatives. The "social fact" was best theorized by the sociologist Émile Durkheim. For Durkheim, to consider society as an object of scientific analysis was to acknowledge it as a reality "exterior to the individual."[6] Science would reveal individualism as nothing more than a moral precept that established a bond of commonality—"humanness"—in complex and diversified modern societies. Individualism, revealed as a product of society and as serving a moral function, could no longer be invoked as a barrier to government-sponsored social reform and intervention. Quite the contrary, Durkheim asserted: The very function of individualism to make people "conscious" of their bonds depended upon the transformation of the state into a moral agent that (through science) would articulate and realize the precepts of human dignity, freedom, and equality. Even as Durkheim employed the "social fact" to legitimize the discipline of sociology, he recognized the importance of hygiene. He referred to the epidemic as pre-eminent proof of the existence of society as a reality exterior to individuals; he adopted etiological analysis as the most effective tool for understanding and regulating that social reality; and his own work drew upon the "moral statistics" that established the authority of hygienists in government circles.[7]

A hygienist as active and influential as Colin would have many opportunities to forge the links between science and politics that produced social facts. Colin was a prolific writer, and his treatises on epidemic disease were crucial to the hygienist's "social" evaluation of Pasteur's theory of germs in the late 1870s and 1880s.[8] That writing earned him a prominent place in the Academy of Medicine and a position as medical inspector in the army. But it was Colin's contribution to the Bureau des épidémies that best exemplifies the constitution of the epidemic as a social fact. The prefect of police established the Bureau des épidémies at the outset of the 1884 cholera outbreak. Administered by a permanent committee of distinguished hygienists that also included Georges Dujardin-Beaumetz and Léon Thoinot, the bureau was charged with finding answers to the long-standing, problematic questions about the origins and transmission of contagious disease, answers made more urgent by the approach of a potentially lethal epidemic. It would obtain this information by verifying each case of contagious disease, and by studying them so as to understand their point of origin and mode of transmission. From the very beginning, however, this process of verification and investigation was implicated in a new regulatory endeavor: Because it was difficult to understand and thus regulate the production of disease in a complex social life like Paris, the only effective strategy was to identify and isolate early cases of disease so as to prevent them from disseminating through the numerous interactions provided by modern city life.

In pursuit of these goals, the bureau created a vast mechanism for collecting information about cases of contagious disease in the city. It appointed medical delegates [médecins délégués] in each of the city's neighborhoods (arrondissements), whose investigations of individual cases were supervised and analyzed by a handful of "medical inspectors"; in addition, the bureau instructed both the long-standing arrondissement hygiene commissions and local police officers to report cases to it. The bureau obtained regular reports from hospitals about patients presumed to have died from contagious disease, and it even depended upon the information-gathering capacities of the rival prefecture of the Seine (in this regard, the Commission on Insalubrious Dwellings and the Municipal Statistical Service were the most important sources of information). Finally, the bureau relied upon letters written by urban residents worried about the possibility of contagious disease in their apartment buildings and neighborhoods. To expedite the speedy transmission of information, the latest technology, including telegraph and (eventually) telephone, was installed. Once collected, the cases of disease were placed upon maps and organized in files according to street and victim's name. That organization facilitated the intimate relationship between explanatory and regulatory goals: Explanations of transmission were formulated, isolation and disinfection services were dispatched, and a way of knowing disease-prone neighborhoods so as to prevent future epidemics was guaranteed.[9]

One of the most important accomplishments of the Bureau des épidémies was the publication of studies of epidemics, also referred to as *enquêtes*, many of which were written or edited by Colin.[10] These publications ranged from lengthy studies of the cholera epidemics of 1884 and 1892 to the annual reports concerning the activities of neighborhood hygiene commissions and the incidence of epidemic (later called contagious) disease in the department of the Seine. Designed to illuminate the elusive social conditions that shaped the operations of contagion in urban life, as well as to evaluate and justify the preventive steps undertaken in conjunction with the collection and analysis of information, the reports also allude to the professional and political interests that constituted knowledge of epidemics as "social fact." The hygienists who wrote and edited these reports invoked both the success and limitations of their explanatory and regulatory efforts to advocate the "unification" and "centralization" of information services at the prefecture of police against the competing claims put forward by the prefect of the Seine. To the extent that unification and centralization of these services under the prefecture of police was demanded as a matter of law, these reports linked the destiny of hygiene's professional power to Republican social reform. A legal recognition of the epidemic service would not only legitimize a regulatory service that was established under the threat of an epidemic and through extraordinary police powers. It would also establish the regulation of disease as central to the efforts of Third Republic politicians to conceive social regulation.

The complex of scientific, professional, and political interests that constituted the epidemic as social fact is best understood by paying attention to the prominent position accorded to the home—*"le foyer"*—in these reports. The home often was the starting point of these administrative efforts to investigate and explain the complex and mysterious patterns of epidemics in urban life. And hygienists ended up defining the home as embodying those various social conditions that were crucial to understanding and regulating contagious disease. In so doing, they were conscious of, and engaged with, the political resonance of the home that had made it an enduring presence in the arena of social regulation throughout the nineteenth century. It is by paying attention to references to the home in these reports that we can understand how decisively the explanation and regulation of contagious disease shaped, and was shaped by, Third Republic social politics.

## The Immigrant and the Origin of Epidemics

"Who can be so deluded so as to believe that he has resolved such a complex problem?" Thus Léon Thoinot modestly began his investigation of the origin of the 1884 cholera epidemic.[11] Thoinot did not offer these words lightly; he had reason to worry. As a chief medical inspector for the recently formed Bureau des épidémies, he took seriously his task to discover how the epidemic developed so swiftly in the departments of southern France. But the cities he was obliged to investigate, Toulon and Marseille, posed only obstacles. Both were large urban agglomerations and active ports that presented myriad opportunities for the importation and precocious transmission of germs. Thoinot could neither isolate the first victim nor discover the link among the first cases in Toulon, nor verify how (or if) the disease had spread from Toulon to Marseille. Thoinot was not alone in the problems he faced. In his presentation of the bureau's official study of the 1892 cholera epidemic in the department of the Seine, Dujardin-Beaumetz found it difficult to connect the first three cases that appeared at the Nanterre shelter, and especially to ascertain whether the disease had been transmitted indirectly by water or through direct human contact.[12] For the leading statistician Jacques Bertillon, the ambiguous and contested diagnostic distinction between cholera *nostras* (an endemic and benign gastro-intestinal disorder characterized by the symptoms of cholera) and cholera *asiatique* (an imported, virulent, and contagious disease) made it impossible for him to confirm the first case of the 1884 epidemic in Paris.[13] And in their investigation of the typhus epidemic that broke out at a night shelter administered by the prefecture of police, Thoinot and his colleague Henri Dubief (also a medical inspector for the bureau) concluded that "no one can be incriminated as having been contaminated."[14]

Despite his initial worries, however, Thoinot did find an explanation for the outbreak of cholera in Toulon: the "immigrant." "The presence of immigrants is the reason for cholera; it is the sole and sufficient reason," was the confident conclusion of this investigator who had begun so hesitantly and who could only make such an assertion by marginalizing other competing factors such as contaminated laundry, water, and merchandise.[15] Thoinot and other bureau investigators employed the category of "immigrant" to explain the origins of epidemics in urban life precisely because it enabled them to surpass the obstacles encountered in a scientific analysis of the origins of epidemics. The extreme mobility that investigators saw as defining the condition of immigrants explained why so many epidemics were characterized by a few disparate and seemingly spontaneous cases, thus making a search for the original case not only impossible but also unnecessary. Because these investigators regarded the immigrant not only as mobile but also as poor and intemperate, that category could bridge the opposing categories of contagious cause and bodily resistance that had fueled debates in the Academy of Medicine and other learned societies. Immigrants could have contracted and spread a virulent germ through the numerous contacts they made in the course of their "vagabondage." Or, more likely, they could have carried a latent germ or come upon a latent germ in urban life that, on account of their depressed resistance created by lack of food and an excess of alcohol, was revived and began a new epidemic outburst. As stated by Auguste Ollivier, a member of the Conseil d'hygiène publique who wrote on the 1893 typhus epidemic, the immigrant conflated many credible scenarios explaining the origin of epidemics in

urban life: "The Paris epidemic demonstrates to us in the most strik-
ing manner the spread [*colportage*] of typhus by vagabonds and the
homeless, exhausted by all kinds of deprivation and offering an easy
prey on account of their wayward life [*hasard de leur vie errante*]."[16]

Even as they relied upon a fixed set of characteristics of immigrant
life to explain the origin of disease in urban life, the variety of social
types they invoked to illuminate the role of the immigrant in disease exposed the category as imprecise. In addition to the more established
and recognizable examples of immigrants—foreigner, vagabond, rag-
picker, and nomad—hygienists identified the student and the sailor
who spread cholera from Toulon to Marseille in 1884,[17] the quarrymen
who facilitated the spread of cholera in the department of the Seine in
1892,[18] as well as the twenty thousand provincials who came to Paris an-
nually in search of work in the "rebuilding of Paris" and ended up creating recurrent typhoid fever epidemics in the 1880s.[19] For hygienists, to
implicate "the immigrant" in the origins of epidemics served to express
anxiety about the inability to know the behavior and whereabouts of so
many, diverse urban inhabitants. Hygienists saw the "anonymity" of
the "immigrant" in urban life as a result of the inadequate mechanisms
of socialization in urban and industrial society. In their view, many urban inhabitants lacked not only the moral, socializing function of the
home. They also escaped those extraordinary policing measures, such as
the inspection of *garnis* and the requirement that visitors present their
passports and workers their *livrets* (work passports) to neighborhood
police commissioners, that were designed to protect urban social order
against what was seen as the destabilizing influence of newcomers and
transients.[20]

Far from bringing a well-defined understanding of the immigrant
to bear upon the obscure problem of the origin of epidemics in urban
life, these investigations served to produce a knowledge of the immigrant and the epidemic relationally. If recourse to what was considered the immigrant's asocial behavior—his or her lack of home life
and the bad habits that followed—explained the origins of disease,
then disease in turn enabled the hygienist to focus on and transform
the understanding of the problem of unsocialized patterns of life in
urban centers. Now associated with the spread of disease, the prob-

lem of socialization that characterized modern urban and industrial centers could neither be analyzed nor resolved through the category of individual liberty. Rather, the lack of social ties and moral capacities represented a danger that would require an extended police regulation of social life. Thus Thoinot wrote in his study of the cholera epidemic that "the foreign choleraic who died was only an illuminating index of the danger which menaces the city, a danger created by the crowds of arriving immigrants."²¹

To convince skeptical readers, Thoinot provided examples, the product of rigorous observation, that portrayed disease as a conflict between the dangers of unsocialized individuals and embattled orderly (because domiciled) residents. "One morning," he wrote, "one of them [Italian immigrants traveling from Marseille to the Drôme] happened to throw up on the doorstep of a home. [The inhabitant] was stricken with cholera, died, and infected [*contagionné*] the entire village."²² Others fashioned the terms of marginal social behavior and social types into etiological categories—"*le colportage de typhus,*" "*une distribution vagabonde*"—in the process giving scientific credence to the dangers posed by unsocialized individuals and thus justifying their regulation.²³ And when attempting to convince readers of the necessity to regulate these dangers, at once epidemiological and social, hygienists foregrounded what urban administrators and members of the general population alike would consider the most threatening of immigrants and the most threatening of spaces: the nomad who sought temporary refuge in the night shelter. In his 1893 report on the night shelters that served as the starting point for the infrequent outbreaks of typhus, Dujardin-Beaumetz focused on this unregulated space that inspires the most "fear":

> · These night shelters, where one does not "go to bed," but where for a small cost of twenty centimes, the price of some soup or a ration of wine, one can spend the night protected and sleep propped up on a table, these establishments whose keepers refuse any [official] visit, any police or hygiene measure applicable to boardinghouses, alleging that they cannot be considered lodging house keepers since in reality they do not have beds, do not offer sleeping facilities to their transient clients and only serve as provisioners of drink [*débitants de boissons*]. There is

no need to insist upon the dangers that, from the viewpoint of the transmission of germs, are provided by these refuges where up to eight or nine hundred people are stuffed.[24]

Hygienists who investigated the origins of epidemics and who wrote these reports were not the first to suggest the role of the immigrant in the origins of disease. The odious (if still invoked) Restoration Law of 1822, which sought to prevent the spread of yellow fever into France by establishing quarantines on the Franco-Spanish border and imposing harsh penalties (including death) on transgressors, was based upon the premise that contagious disease was imported.[25] Unlike Restoration officials, however, late-nineteenth-century hygienists saw the immigrant's role in disease as created by, rather than imposed upon, French society. Despite its claim to "close Paris to the transient poor,"[26] Haussmann's rebuilding of Paris had facilitated the influx of people in search of work and pleasure and unacclimated to the rigors of urban life; it had expanded (or did not prevent the expansion of) night shelters throughout the city; it had created the cafés, theaters, and (above all) boulevards where newcomers both contracted and transmitted disease; and it had abandoned the housing problem to the vicissitudes of the free market, thus depriving many of the newly arrived working poor of the moral, socializing influences of the home.[27]

Hygienists indicated how their understanding of the immigrant was shaped by political questions about the future possibilities of social regulation. Even when hygienists could confirm with relative certainty the importation of disease from a foreign boat harbored in a French port, they nonetheless continued to emphasize the social conditions that had established the immigrant as the origin of disease.[28] In justifying this position, hygienists argued that the regulatory practices that followed from a recognition of importation—especially quarantine—were from "another epoch," the repressive age of the Restoration. Meanwhile, a focus on the social conditions of immigrant life enabled them to address the shortcomings of the social politics of Haussmannization. In their view, the role of the immigrant in the origins of disease revealed Haussmannization—despite its professed goals—as insufficiently social. One of the professed goals of Haussmannization was to "solidify family organization within the city."[29] But the commitment of the Second Empire to speculative practices (which that regime shared with its Republican adversaries) limited its intervention in the construction and improvement of housing for the working poor, "sacrificed" the home to the embellishment of the street and other public places, and thereby demonstrated (in the view of hygienists) the incompatibility of the values of private property and the moral function of the home. Even the Second Empire's limited experiment with "assistance" failed to inculcate any feelings of social duty on the part of the recipient; "nomads" and "mendicants" paid for the "hospitality" of shelter by spreading cholera.[30] For hygienists, to situate the "immigrant" origin of disease in society was to engage in the politics of social regulation from which they had largely been excluded: to pursue, through the association of disease and the home, the regulation of a social interest that avoided the equally ineffective alternatives of repression and nonintervention adopted by past regimes.

### The Foyer and the Transmission of Disease

By implicating society in the possibilities of disease, the focus on the "immigrant" led hygienists to subordinate a consideration of the origin of disease (which had assumed such a prominent position in Pasteurian investigations of disease) to the explanation of the development and spread of disease. Here, hygienists confronted new obstacles. Hygienists were struck by the "unequal" distribution of cases in the city. Conscious of the political resonance carried by such an analytical term, they quickly pointed out that the observation of unequal distribution could not be understood as the expression of the opposing conditions of rich and poor arrondissements. Sometimes the wealthy neighborhoods of western Paris produced disease. More problematically, they observed that within the poorer arrondissements of Paris, epidemic disease appeared to favor specific streets, clusters of apartment buildings, and even individual dwellings, always accompanied by sporadic cases that radiated out of these clusters—or what hygienists began to describe as *foyers* of disease.[31]

We have already seen how observations such as these fueled scientific debates over the relative merits of a contagious cause and physiological processes in the production of disease. This was especially true for investigations of typhoid fever and cholera, the two diseases that received the most attention at the height of the Pasteurian debates in the 1880s. For Martellière, the *rapporteur* for the Second Arrondissement Hygiene Commission, *foyers* of typhoid fever presented two characteristics that could not be explained by an exclusive recourse to either infection or contagion. First, Martellière addressed the question of the permanence of the *foyer*:

> It is a question of knowing when a disease is fixed for a period of time in a neighborhood, in a circumscribed area, if it stays there permanently in specific homes, infecting the inhabitants successively, or if it propagates gradually. . . . When an interval of only two or three months passes between successive cases, the hypothesis of direct transmission is possible; but with an interval of fifteen or twenty months, many times confirmed, it is no longer possible to establish a filiation.[32]

Martellière illuminated such ruminations with many specific examples including the case of a young girl who was the sole member of her family to contract typhoid fever; ten months later her younger sister was stricken and died. Was this a case of direct transmission between two siblings facilitated by the "lodging itself," Martellière wondered? Did the sisters contract the disease coincidentally from one of the many "indirect" sources of contagion that existed in these apartment buildings (a badly sealed cesspool, a neighbor's cesspool, a water supply that, however repulsive, is used to clean vegetables and dishes)? Or was the second death due to a change in the banal conditions of the home that had earlier enabled other family members to resist the transmission of disease (he verified that the single room the family occupied was, at the time of the first death, vast, healthy, and sunny)? If so, how might one reconcile such a role for the home with the mechanism of contagion?[33] The question of the distance between the two deaths brought Martellière to introduce the second troubling

characteristic of the *foyer*, the selectivity of victims within a circum-
scribed, constant area of disease. "When one examines the distribution of typhoid fever in detail, one sees the illness affect a certain
number of inhabitants, while excluding ten, twenty others who by all
rights should have contracted the disease."[34]

In the august setting of the Academy of Medicine, questions such
as these surfaced around the 1884 cholera epidemic, making it one of
the most intensively studied and contested (if least lethal) epidemics
of the century.[35] Guérin used the observed combination of concentrated and dispersed cases of cholera to prove his theory that the disease began spontaneously under banal conditions, only later to become contagious. Dujardin-Beaumetz blamed the transmission of
cholera on direct contagion within families, yet not without recognizing that the stricken families' reputation for drunkenness also suggested the importance of receptivity. Colin indicted rag-pickers for
the cases of cholera he observed in the suburb of St. Ouen.[36] Some
saw these *foyers* as spreading disease to the surrounding lodgings and
apartment buildings (even apparently salubrious ones), while others
identified them as constituting true *îlots* of disease. Academy member
Hardy recognized in these contradictory explanations a definite incapacity of expert observation to explain the mechanism behind the
creation of the *foyer*, and he cautioned the academy against invoking
that category to legitimize controversial measures to combat cholera,
such as government intervention in the home.[37] Meanwhile, Brouardel (as always) tried to reconcile these diverse findings by noting that
insalubriousness was a necessary but insufficient condition of disease,
which could not be produced without the transmission of a germ.

In the context of these scientific difficulties and the volatile political and professional interests they inevitably raised, hygienists transformed the *foyer* from a descriptive into an explanatory category.
Whereas it originally served to express the inexplicable presence in
urban life of permanent and concentrated pockets of disease surrounded by sporadic cases, the *foyer* now explained how the home
caused disease transmission in a way that brought together the contested categories of infection and contagion. Both the individuals and
the physical structures (toilets, courtyards, kitchens, water supplies)

that composed these homes could spread disease through direct and indirect contagion between family members, other families who resided in the apartment building, and beyond. Germs that existed permanently in these homes in latent form could be revived by a change in the banal conditions of both the infected home and the surrounding lodgings.

Hygienists reconciled these many alternatives with their goal to establish a simple etiology of disease by defining individual moral comportment as the factor that constituted a *foyer* of disease. Whether created by direct or indirect transmission of a germ, or by a change in the conditions of the home that revived a latent germ or made residents susceptible to disease, hygienists reduced the problem of the *foyer* to a function of social practices. According to Dubief, if working-class children could contract scarlet fever in a number of places—the public spaces of apartment buildings, in public gardens, or on the street—the disease was due, above all, to mothers who worked outside the home and thus could not adequately *"surveille"* them.[38] Commenting upon the smallpox epidemic that emerged in 1882 in the thirteenth arrondissement, the mayor and *rapporteur* for the neighborhood hygiene commission argued that "a regular life, a rigorous cleaning of body and dwelling, are the best preservatives against all diseases and especially epidemic ones."[39] Dr. Martellière did not resolve the debate over whether human waste left in ill-equipped toilets, apartment corridors, or sewers was the source of typhoid fever, but instead focused on waste "that one has not disinfected."[40] In his 1884 investigation of the cholera epidemic, Thoinot used notions of ignorance and negligence to fashion into a simple etiology the various conditions of the home, from transmission to uncleanliness, that he saw as causing that epidemic:

> Here, for example, is a family composed of five or six poor people igno-
> rant of the basic rules of hygiene. The family inhabits one or two rooms
> into which it is crowded. One of the members is stricken with a disease;
> what are the chances that the others will not be infected? The excrement
> of the stricken individual will be thrown here and there in the room or
> left without any precaution in a jar, consequently corrupting the already
> insufficient air of the house. The linens, the bedsheets will be sullied and

handled by everyone; the contagion will thus be direct, or will happen indirectly through the contamination of food that came in contact with sullied hands.[41]

In a report produced by the Conseil d'hygiène publique on a diphtheria epidemic at a school on the rue François Miron, Ollivier put the matter more simply: "I have said it before and I will repeat it every chance I get: The two principal factors of the diffusion of diphtheria, like all the other epidemic diseases that afflict the indigent, are ignorance and negligence."[42]

In reducing the complex and sometimes contested role of the home to social practices, hygienists demonstrated how profoundly their investigations and attempts at explanation were shaped by the regulatory meanings associated with the term *foyer*. In Republican discourse, the *foyer* represented the home as fostering those human moral and social capacities that made it possible to conceive of a free social order. Grounded in "sexual difference," in the notion that women's nature made them at once suited for moral tasks and incapable of exercising reason and enjoying rights, the *foyer* gave expression to anxiety about the potential of the Revolutionary promise of individual liberty to create the conditions for social order.

The hygienist's conception of *foyer* aimed at offering a new resolution of the conflict between the free individual and social order, liberty and sociability, by posing them as distinct and sometimes opposing capacities. This was best articulated by Henri Monod, the prefect of the department of the Finistère (in the Brittany region of France) whose lengthy *enquête* on the cholera epidemic there in 1885 would establish his credentials as the future minister of assistance. Monod argued that the *foyer* of disease "puts into evidence with increasing precision and certainty the laws of solidarity. From then on, new duties have appeared." Republican legislators and academics coined the term solidarism to reassert the inextricable relationship between individual liberty and moral duty as a justification for the Republic's obligation to pursue limited economic and social reform. For Monod, however, the laws of solidarity as revealed by the *foyer* suggested only the dangers that the actions of free individuals—here understood as the enjoyment of property and privacy—posed for social order. Monod observed that "one knows that the insalubriousness of the home does not only endanger those who inhabit it, but that this home is destined to become the *foyer* of an epidemic which will spread afar."[43] The lesson to be drawn from this understanding of the *foyer* was regulatory: the obligation of government, in the social interest of preventing disease, to intervene in what was once considered the inviolable sphere of free, self-regulating individuals, in order to repress those dangerous moral and social practices of free individuals, as well as to encourage salutary ones. "Society should not remain unarmed against such dangers," urged the mayor and *rapporteur* for the eleventh arrondissement hygiene commission in 1881, a year that witnessed a resurgence of smallpox in Paris.[44]

In their attempt to fashion the *foyer* as the basis for a new vision of society that depended upon the regulatory force of government, and not individual liberty, hygienists forged links with investigations of an earlier age written by (among others) Villermé, Buret, and Frégier. Like their famous predecessors, late-nineteenth-century hygienists included among the dangers to be indicted and regulated dissipated and drunken male workers who wasted time and money at cafés, single women who worked rather than assume the duties of marriage and motherhood, and mothers who neglected their children by accepting industrial work outside of the home. While members of an earlier generation had attempted to square their observations and prescriptions with a continued commitment to the principle of individual liberty, in the process undermining the scientific credibility and power of their work, late-nineteenth-century hygienists invoked the objectivity of their findings as sufficient grounds for accepting a new understanding of society that would entail regulating the home. An investigation into tuberculosis undertaken by the Academy of Medicine simply posited contrasting evidence to prove the danger of women who lived outside monogamous family relations: Three apprentice seamstresses who shared a bed with their *patronne* ended up dying of tuberculosis, while the three families they had left in search of work presented no indication of disease.[45] And Thoinot's zealous and gratuitous attention to the facts of differential reception of cholera in a closed setting itself contained a judgment upon women who did not take seriously their familial duties:

> Mrs. R., . . . , who was the first to die of cholera in this town, arrived there experiencing the symptoms of diarrhea. She entered a hotel, spent the night with her lover who did not refrain from holding her in his arms, and who had sexual relations with her while the symptoms of cholera were evident, kissed her on the mouth between her bouts of vomiting. Mrs. R. was rushed to the hospital and died there; her lover remained immune.[46]

Even as hygienists relied upon scientific objectivity to express judgments about "dangerous" social practices and to propose controversial social prescriptions entailing government intervention in the home, they demonstrated how decisively professional and political interests had shaped these "social facts." Hygienists who pursued their investigations under the auspices of the prefect of police often apostrophized "observation" as the authority that would expose and resolve the problems of Haussmannization, in the process securing their tenuous position in the contested realm of social regulation. Thus, according to the *rapporteur* of the hygiene commission of the nineteenth arrondissement,

> [s]ome years after the promulgation of the law, the transformation of Paris began; after forty years of trial, observation wonders if this transformation was a good thing. Certainly the wide, spacious boulevards are a benefit; the demolition of old homes is an auspicious result, but the hygienist penetrates further and states painfully that the inhabitants of the rue de Rivoli have less air and light than those on the rue Vieille-du-Temple, for example.[47]

The prefect of the Seine responded to these scientific assertions of police authority by creating under his jurisdiction new mechanisms and offices devoted to the investigation of disease. In doing so, both prefectures accepted the political (discursive) operations of scientific objectivity: to remove the possibilities of social order from the contested category of liberty by transforming the social and moral practices of home life into an object of knowledge and regulation.

## The Public Health Law of 1902

These investigations, focused on the pre-eminent, capital city of France and undertaken by hygienists of national and international renown, could not help but resonate with social interests and regulatory concerns that extended well beyond the problem of socialization in Paris. Indeed, hygienists moved effortlessly between the issues of Paris and national ones. Sounding a "cry of alarm" in the 1880s, they placed their social facts in the service of the populationist debate that preoccupied the fledgling Republic in the decades following the Franco-Prussian War.[48] France, hygienists pointed out, suffered a disproportionately high number of deaths from diseases like typhoid fever and tuberculosis. A nation that realized population increase only through immigration could no longer allow so many young people to die before they had a chance to start a family. In a world where population was regarded as contributing to national strength, a comparison of smallpox statistics proved sobering. Fewer than 400 Prussian troops succumbed to smallpox, while 23,400 French soldiers had died from that disease; in 1870–81, 200,000 French had died from smallpox, equivalent to the number of French soldiers killed in battle. For hygienists, these lamentable statistics had everything to do with France's inadequate regulation. Smallpox was a preventable disease, as Prussia's policy of obligatory vaccination (and France's refusal to do so) amply proved. Hygienists did not hesitate to point out that England, Italy, Sweden, and Belgium had established more comprehensive regulatory systems than France. What made this situation all the more intolerable, in their estimation, was that such regulatory inadequacies existed in a nation renowned for scientific innovation and accomplishment, the very nation that had produced Pasteur.[49]

To address these problems, hygienists called for the creation of a national public health (hygiene) administration authorized to identify, investigate, and regulate the *foyers* that spread disease.[50] Hygienists, now associated with renovated (that is, fully and legally empowered) departmental hygiene councils, would institute a permanent *enquête* to identify *foyers*, prohibit the habitation of dwellings deemed insalubrious until adequate disinfection procedures had been completed, ensure the expropriation of those dwellings judged permanently insalubrious, as well as write and implement guidelines for the construction of new, salubrious dwellings. While some of these proposals had already been realized through administrative decree or the exercise of extraordinary police powers (the Bureau des épidémies is a good example of this), hygienists sought legitimacy for disease regulation in the new Republican order that only "the law" could provide. Hygienists appreciated the unique status of law among the regulatory instruments employed in a Republican social order.[51] The Republican vision of law was premised upon a recognition of the free individual as essentially self-regulating; in accordance with this vision, legal regulation was limited mainly to the intermittent repression of threats to the exercise of individual liberty. Hygienists understood that such a narrow conception of law in the past had limited their efforts to eliminate and prevent the social conditions that produced disease. In proposing a new and extended regulation of disease, at once consistent, permanent, prescriptive, and focused on the home, as a matter of a public health *law*, hygienists sought nothing less than to redefine the very possibilities of a free social order. Henceforth, so they hoped, liberty would be premised upon a larger social interest, which could be developed and defended only through an expanded practice of government regulation. Such a new understanding of the relationship between liberty and social order as the basis for a public health law, Monod argued, would establish liberty and regulation not as antagonistic forces, but as mutually reinforcing ones: "[A] law that protects the public health, if wisely conceived, conforms to, and does not contradict, the true principles of liberty."[52]

Ever since the passage of the ill-fated Law of 1850, hygienists had called upon government to address its inadequacies. But it was not until the conjuncture that realized the ascendancy of hygiene and Republicanism in the 1880s that such a reconsideration began in earnest. Which is not to say that it proceeded smoothly or swiftly. Propositions to reform the Law of 1850 were introduced into the Chamber of Deputies in 1881, 1886, 1887, and 1889. Most of these proposals confirmed the framework and spirit of the 1850 law rather than to adopt regulatory innovations grounded in the changing scientific understandings of disease. The Société de médecine publique drafted an official report for the chamber in 1882 that endorsed either a radical transformation or replacement of the 1850 law; and in 1884 the Comité consultatif d'hygiène publique began to draft a government-sponsored project of law that was deposed before the chamber in 1892 and reported in 1893. Two years later, the chamber approved the bill and sent it on to the senate. More conservative than the chamber in matters of social reform, the senate after much delay deliberated the law on three separate occasions between 1897 and 1901. It returned a radically scaled back law to the chamber in 1901, and the law was not voted until 1902.[53]

Historians have generally agreed that the long gestation and transformation of this proposed law was the result of a conflict between the scientific claims of hygienists who sought to regulate the insalubrious home as the origin of epidemics and politicians who found such a proposed regulation an unacceptable infringement on liberty, the rights to property and privacy.[54] Given the complex interests that produced the epidemic and the *foyer* as "social fact," it is perhaps more useful to see the arduous battles that emerged in discussions of the law as a conflict between two different political visions about the relationship between liberty and social regulation.

Deputies and senators who opposed the bill grounded their arguments in scientific considerations, questioning the rigor of the hygienist's conception of the *foyer* that lay at the heart of the proposed legislation. They addressed the contradictory evidence about the transmission of cholera and exposed the many, sometimes hidden, variables that were obscured by (in their estimation) this all too perfunctory category. Senator Treille focused on hygienists' understanding of typhoid fever, and concluded that they relied too heavily upon this one disease in the formulation of legislation aiming at the regulation of so many contagious diseases.[55] Having put into question the scientific certainty of hygienists' pronouncements, opponents could more powerfully reveal the political stakes involved in the hygienists' proposal to legislate a regulation of the home. Senator Volland, a severe and convincing critic of the bill, warned his credulous colleagues that the "scientific" understanding of the *foyer* was nothing more than a "pretext" for the consolidation of state power against the prerogatives of individual liberty.

> Would you not fear, as a result of the hygiene laws you vote today, of having armed the representatives of the state with the right to enter (*pénétrer*) whenever they want, on an order issued in Paris, outside of established guarantees of justice, day or night, inside our homes . . . , to come into our homes in order to wage war on microbes and, under the pretext of searching for microbes or infection, open up our most private possessions and our drawers?[56]

Volland and other critics identified three ways in which the hygienists' attempt to explain and regulate contagious disease would increase state power at the expense of liberty. First, it would drastically and unnecessarily curtail the enjoyment of property. The law as supported by hygienists sought to punish the property owner, by prescribing improvements to be made or by expropriation, for causes of insalubriousness that were often uncertain and unattributable. Even in the presence of such causes, these critics wondered, could the state invoke the danger of disease to prescribe and enforce how the home should be "inhabited and maintained"?[57] In the name of protecting society against those infected homes that spread disease, critics contended, the state also sought to deny the right to communal liberty that the Third Republic had so recently reaffirmed in the Municipality Law of 1884. Again, Volland summarized the objection most eloquently: "It is we, sirs, in an era of democracy, who are going to remove from our laws an essential democratic principle, the guarantee and control offered to us by an elected (municipal) official."[58] For Volland and others, a law that made the deliberations of a municipal council accountable to the expert judgments of state-appointed hygienists would completely negate the "public law" that formed the very foundation of the Republic. Thus Senator Milliès-Lacroix felt compelled to oppose the proposition of law, not because he did not appreciate the benefits of ensuring hygiene and public health, but because he maintained "municipalities can take care of the interests which are entrusted to them."[59]

Finally, what made this subordination of communal autonomy to the state and its agents even more odious was the unprecedented concentration of power the bill accorded to hygienists, which was seen as violating the principle of separation of powers. As advisors to the government, hygienists proposed the regulations to be legislated. In fulfillment of their duties as members of the departmental (prefectoral) hygiene councils, they would also administer prescriptions, judge their validity, and evaluate the legitimacy of appeals filed by property owners who protested the imposition of fines and expropriation. "Why, because it is a question of hygiene," Volland asked, "are we for example going to confound the domains which must never be merged or confounded? Why are we going to merge the judiciary with the administration?"[60]

Defenders of the proposed legislation addressed these criticisms through a continued adherence to the besieged dichotomy between science and politics. Taudrière, the chamber's most spirited defender of the bill, argued that the identification and regulation of a home as a *foyer* of disease made questions of communal and individual rights irrelevant. As an embodiment of "danger," the regulation of the *foyer* involved a different interest and a different jurisdiction; it posed a threat to society and could be addressed only through hygienic expertise.[61] In this view, a review undertaken by the nation's highest administrative court, the Conseil d'état, would be incompetent to judge the merits of hygienists' findings and prescriptions; it could merely ensure that they were adequately observed and implemented. When critics, continuing their efforts to expose the political interests that informed science, asked their colleague what constituted a *foyer*, or "[w]hat constitutes a building which cannot be sanitized [*assaini*]," Taudrière responded: "It's not I who can respond to a question concerning hygiene."[62] He then referred such questions to Brouardel who, as president of the Comité consultatif d'hygiène publique, attended these legislative debates in an advisory capacity.

In this setting, Brouardel wonderfully represented the independence of scientific objectivity from political considerations. Responding to concerns that the judgments of hygienists would interfere with the enjoyment of property and the exercise of communal and individual rights, Brouardel modestly recognized his lack of competence to comment upon judicial matters before the chamber. Consequently, he could assure its members that hygienists were not "tyrannical" and maintained no agenda to "judge the right of property"; in any event, all of their decisions would be liable to regulation by the prefects and the minister of the interior.[63] But just as hygienists were both ill equipped and disinclined to participate in judicial and political decisions, so too in his view municipal councils lacked the scientific expertise required to evaluate and regulate insalubrious housing. For those opponents skeptical of his insistence on hygienic competence, Brouardel offered sobering statistics that indicted the principle of self-regulation in matters of disease: "In 1887–88, in the arrondissement of Pontivy, out of a total of 110,000 inhabitants, there were 1,034 deaths from smallpox; in Douarnenez, out of 10,900 inhabitants, there were 844 deaths from smallpox, that is nearly 1 in 10. . . ." And in response to Volland, who had used the experience of the Commission on Insalubrious Dwellings in his hometown of Nancy to justify his continued support of a law that affirmed communal self-regulation, Brouardel did not hesitate to point out that Nancy possessed a higher mortality rate than the national average, 26.5/1,000 compared with 23/1,000.[64]

Despite this masterful presentation, however, Brouardel could not completely dissociate his representation of science from a statist vision of social regulation that his opponents claimed was at the basis of this proposal of law. He argued that the regulation of disease crystallized a national interest and thus needed to be recognized as an *"oeuvre d'état."* In response to those critics who sought to legislate disease regulation as a matter of communal autonomy, he spoke of the "tyranny" of local authority.[65] (Paul Strauss, who had not yet joined the senate at the time of these debates but who as a member of the Paris Municipal Council—and the future founding minister of hygiene, assistance and social welfare—vigorously supported the legislation, likewise worried about the *"anarchie sanitaire"* that would ensue if the regulation of disease was left to the commune and the city.)[66] More problematically, Brouardel and others, in an attempt to diffuse the charge that the proposed regulation of the home would serve the interests of state power at the expense of liberty, identified other, more palatable political motives that informed the law. In an allusion to the spirit of the 1850 law that the danger of the *foyer* was intended to invalidate, Brouardel urged skeptical senators to think of the suffering poor who would benefit from regulations concerning insalubrious housing.[67] Senator Cordelet asked his colleagues not to regard the proposed law as an innovation but rather as a revision of the 1850 law. And Monod, who attended these debates as a government advisor [*"commissaire du gouvernement"*] and who had in other circumstances celebrated the innovative character of the law, here attempted to assuage senators by presenting the regulatory provisions of the law as based upon the principle of individual rights. "This is a new application of a principle as old as society itself, to wit that no one has the right to harm another," he stated reassuringly.[68] This introduction of new principles was not rhetorical, but rather was accompanied by the efforts of hygienists and their supporters to modify the regulatory power proposed by the bill. The law, they argued, would not create hygiene as an independent jurisdiction with the authority to pronounce, execute, and evaluate judgments concerning insalubrious dwellings. Rather, the departmental councils would depend upon mayors to execute judgments by issuing decrees [*arrêtés*], and they would serve only at the discretion of their respective prefects.

It was the highly politicized question of regulation that accounts for the bizarre law that was finally voted in 1902.[69] At the conceptual center of the law was the *foyer*, the insalubrious home that threatened society and that government, in the interest of society, was obliged to regulate. It no longer mattered, as had been the case with the Insalubrious Dwellings Law of 1850, whether the causes of insalubriousness were permanent (structural) or the result of the enjoyment of the occupant, whether the home was inhabited by the owner or a tenant, or whether tenants or investigating hygienists had brought insalubrious conditions to the attention of regulatory authorities. Instead, the law articulated a single criterion: "It suffices that [the dwelling] pose a danger to neighbors."[70] The law confirmed the obligatory declaration of cases of contagious diseases as originally stated in the 1892 law regarding the medical profession.[71] It extended this regulatory function of information by empowering prefects to undertake an *enquête* in any commune or city in their respective jurisdictions with rates of disease above the national average. Finally, it required every commune to adopt a comprehensive "sanitary regulation" and every city with a population of more than twenty thousand to establish a hygiene bureau.

These provisions suggest that the 1902 law created through science a new kind of social regulation—consistent (as opposed to intermittent) and prescriptive (and not repressive)—that had made disease regulation such an intensely politicized topic since the 1832 cholera epidemic. The law, however, contained one fatal flaw: It failed to create a regulatory power—an *"assainissement d'office"*—adequate to realizing the positive, daily social intervention demanded by legislators and hygienists.[72] By empowering the communal mayors, whose interests were aligned more closely with the municipal council than with the state, to create and execute sanitary regulation, the law ended up affirming individual and communal liberty as the source of social regulation. The authority of the prefectoral hygiene councils to approve the "sanitary regulation" did not differ significantly from the advisory role originally accorded to them in the largely ineffective 1848 decree, while the ability of prefects to intervene when mayors proved ineffective simply confirmed the intermittent use of police powers established by the 1790 Law on Municipalities.

Given the influential role of *enquêtes* undertaken by the Conseil d'hygiène publique, it is worth considering this problem of *exécution d'office* as it pertained to the regulation of disease in the department of the Seine. A 1903 law that addressed the "unique" requirements of the capital department affirmed the status quo that split the regulation of disease between the prefects of the Seine and police. While the law extended the jurisdiction of the prefect of the Seine over the contested "shared" spaces in apartment buildings—passageways, corridors, communal toilets—it also recognized the long-standing authority of the prefect of police to collect information and regulate cases of contagious disease, to regulate boardinghouses [*garnis*], as well as to formulate and enforce measures for vaccination and disinfection (which the prefect of the Seine, in turn, would "administer," or implement). In refusing the demand that the prefect of police become the basis for a new, enlarged, and positive regulation of disease, senators and deputies sought to limit an authority whose history was bound up with the repression of Republicanism. Thus, in an 1887 report, the legislator Chautemps exclaimed that "[a] prefect of police does not concern himself with microbes; he is preoccupied only with red flags and seditious symbols. . . ."[73] By refusing to transform or dismantle that office in favor of the prefect of the Seine, however, legislators confessed their inability or unwillingness to conceive of state power in a Republican social order beyond such an intermittent use of repressive force.

For all of its shortcomings, however, the Public Health Law of 1902 did not simply reconfirm the regulatory inadequacies of 1850. Rather, it revealed the tactical error of hygienists and their advocates who sought to legislate social regulation. That goal failed to take into account how, in Revolutionary France, "the law" had come to be defined in terms of a conception and practice of liberty that could conceive of state regulation only negatively. Strauss expressed succinctly how heavily the Revolution weighed upon this failed attempt to legislate a new kind of social regulation: "It is always dangerous," he said, "to tamper with legislation dating from Messidor An VIII."[74] In the end, the real innovation of hygienists would be not to legislate a positive social regulation, but to realize such a regulation outside the sphere of legislation.

## CHAPTER 5

# Hygienic Observation and the Remaking of Police Regulation

## I. Introduction: The Limits of Law

Historians are unanimous in their acceptance of the Public Health Law of 1902 as the endpoint and defining moment of the century-long preoccupation with contagious disease. They disagree, however, on both the effectiveness of the law and its larger political, social, and scientific significance. In a recent and important collection on the "Pasteurian Revolution" edited by the French historian of science Claire Salomon-Bayet, Robert Carvais argued that the Public Health Law of 1902 represented an acknowledgment, however tardy, of the Republic's commitment to "social rights," realized here in the "right to health":

> After "a century of relative immobility," the laws started to proliferate at the dawn of the twentieth century and constituted a coherent right to health, aided in this by authors, legislators convinced of the beneficial aspect of Pasteurism. ... This right of the inviolable human body, a principle of civil law, comes up against the constraints posed by the public health. Between an individual liberty and a collective obligation, the choice is made in favor of the latter.[1]

Not all historians have offered such optimistic interpretations, however. Lion Murard and Patrick Zylberman have emphasized the limited regulatory powers of the law, which they regard as a product of the failure of statist hygienists and their political allies to prepare the "manners and customs" (*moeurs*) of free French citizens for such an invasive intervention in private life. Ann-Louise Shapiro's more materialist interpretation indicts the role of bourgeois interests—most importantly limited government, the inviolability of the "private sphere," and private property—in limiting the claims of science for a legislated regulation of the home. "In examining the legislation of 1902," she argued, "it seemed clear that, in the end, the priorities of the legislators determined the parameters within which reform could occur. Where hygienists seemed to challenge long-standing assumptions about private property and political authority, legislators resisted innovation."[2]

My objective is not to judge the relative merits of either side of this interpretive debate (both positions, as the preceding chapter suggests, contain valid points). Rather, I want to question the necessity of adopting the 1902 law, and "the rule of law" more generally, as the vantage point from which to evaluate nineteenth-century efforts to regulate disease. In relying upon this law, historians have uncritically accepted the "symbiosis" between law and science that occupied such a prominent position in Republican discourse.[3] This symbiosis defined social regulation as an expression of individual liberty and rights, an expression revealed and guaranteed by the exercise of human reason that was taken to be the common characteristic of science and law and the basis for their collaboration. The "symbiosis" between law and science, while appealing, oversimplifies the relationship between science and social regulation. It acknowledges neither the deeply contested political issues concerning the relationship between individual liberty and social regulation that shaped the process of scientific knowledge about disease nor the innovative (and unexpected) ways of thinking about and regulating social life that resulted from such a process.[4]

Late-nineteenth-century hygienists, good Republicans that they were, drew upon this vision of the symbiotic relationship between law and science in their attempts to understand and regulate disease, yet not without suspecting its inadequacies. Their doubts concerning a legal regulation of disease became manifest during what we have already seen to be a defining moment in the development of nineteenth-century disease regulation: the cholera epidemic of 1884. Official investigations and debates at the outset of the epidemic and afterward focused on the problem of the *porteur des germes*—of individuals who unknowingly carry and transmit latent germs that serve as the origin of epidemic outbursts. The problems raised by the latent carrier were at once scientific and political. For Brouardel, who as a member of the national Cholera Commission was sent to Toulon to investigate the origin of the disease on French territory so as to prevent its spread to Paris, the lack of symptoms made it impossible to identify and regulate the carrier of a latent germ. Disinfection points at the borders, hospital isolation, and quarantine all appeared inadequate from a scientific point of view. These difficulties were aggravated by the character of social life, which not only provided numerous opportunities for transmitting and (of more serious concern for Paris-oriented investigators) "exporting" disease but also guaranteed the anonymity of infected people. It was the obstacles provided by the recognition of the *porteur* that account for the sobering conclusion of the commission report written by Brouardel:

> [O]ne does not leave a contaminated city only by train. In Toulon, long lines of carts, carrying bags and runaways, followed one another on the roads. . . . Will it be necessary to establish lazarettos on all the train, land, and water routes with the objective of allowing to elapse the period of possible incubation, in which separations are made to isolate travelers by groups according to observation dates? The commission was not able to give its support to these illusory measures, which only have the appearance of hygiene, [but] which really compromise it by inspiring a false sense of security.[5]

In subsequent discussions of this report that took place at the Comité consultatif d'hygiène, the Academy of Medicine, and the Société de médecine publique, it became clear that hygienists were not simply concerned with the possible ineffectiveness of regulating asymptomatic carriers through the practices of disinfection, isolation, and quarantine. Of greater concern was whether the adoption and implementation of such measures, even if effective, would violate long-standing Republican principles. In the view of hygienists, regulatory strategies like quarantines, requiring travelers to register with police authorities, placing individuals in disinfection boxes (a practice adopted in both Belgium and Austria), and hospital isolation wards were problematic not only because the nature of the *porteur* rendered them "illusory" from a scientific viewpoint. They also offended the political sensibilities of hygienists whose faith in the capacity of science to regulate disease was conceived within the Republican parameters of a government respectful of individual rights and the rule of law. Charles Daremberg, the Sorbonne historian of medicine whose massive *Histoire des sciences médicales* charted the development of medical knowledge as an index of the progress of civilization, claimed to have experienced a maritime quarantine in the past and was now not afraid to admit that he preferred cholera to the "suppression" of the "life of nations."[6]

Brouardel, who had written the report suggesting the ineffectiveness of both traditional and innovative (that is, Pasteurian) regulatory measures, resisted Daremberg's depiction of regulation and Republicanism as mutually exclusive goals. True, Brouardel admitted, at present adequate regulatory measures appeared elusive. In the meantime, however, he advocated the legal establishment of a national hygienic administration that would seek out information about dwellings where cases of contagious disease had occurred. Such a service would not only further knowledge about the operations of the *porteur* and how to effectively regulate it; the service would also be a model for regulation worthy of Republicanism. Thus he justified it at a meeting of the Academy of Medicine:

> It is not a question of placing at its head an autocrat imposing his law; but one must recognize that an effective authority is necessary. Let us take for example the Law of 1850 on Insalubrious Dwellings; the commissions designated by this law have only an advisory role; it is easy for a property owner to refuse to remove a cause of insalubriousness in his building. . . . It is not enough to establish that a house is insalubrious, it is necessary to sanitize it.[7]

Brouardel's optimistic pronouncement, however, was riddled with an immense contradiction. He could only conceive of a legal regulation of contagious disease negatively, as an enterprise that would avoid repression (like the Law of 1822) and impotent conciliation (like the Law of 1850). Although he articulated his faith that a scientific regulation of disease based upon the collection and analysis of knowledge about cases of disease and the dwellings in which they occurred could be developed within the parameters of law, he was incapable of addressing (or unwilling to address) the problems that had hindered, since 1850, the attempt to legislate such a regulation of disease: How would municipal or state government find out about individual cases of disease? How would they require the disinfection of private property and the isolation of victims? Standing between Brouardel's optimism and the establishment of a legally sanctioned regulation of disease was the Republican principle of individual liberty, manifested in claims about property rights and the inviolability of family life. In the end, the inability to articulate a regulatory strategy created an atmosphere in these official hygiene venues that is best described as uncomprehending, even desperate. Paul Strauss, the Paris municipal councilor who in another context declared that "[s]ince the Pasteurian revolution, public hygiene moves to assume its deserved place in the government of populations and the administration of cities," displayed naive obstinacy at the discussion of the Société de médecine publique. "It is impossible," he declared, "that this discussion end without a practical solution." Durand-Claye, the eminent engineer associated with the administration of the model Paris sewer system, appeared equally incredulous during the same discussion: "Is there not then any way of protecting [from cholera] the two million human beings crowded into Paris? Are we absolutely defenseless?"[8]

Something approaching Brouardel's vision, however, did emerge out of the 1884 epidemic: the Bureau des épidémies, which was established under the auspices of the prefecture of police and reorganized in 1892 as the Service des épidémies. The bureau took as its primary objective the investigation of *foyers* of disease. Like Brouardel, members and advocates of the bureau appreciated the regulatory power of the law; they sought to legitimize the bureau's practice of a regular and prescriptive intervention in the home as consistent with the Republican value of individual liberty through its inclusion in a broader public health legislation. As we have seen, such a quest largely failed. But in identifying the law as a source of legitimacy for their efforts, bureau members materialized the professional and political interests that produced the symbiotic relationship between law and science thus made it possible to conceive differently the role of science in the creation of social regulation. Here, the impressive activity of the bureau prior to the passage of the 1902 law is instructive: It developed a conception and practice of social regulation through what is best described as the symbiosis between science and policing. In this chapter, I want to consider the development and functioning of this symbiosis from the vantage point of one specific component of disease regulation, the Paris neighborhood (arrondissement) hygiene commissions.

## II. Les commissions d'hygiène d'arrondissement

The prefect of police created the neighborhood commissions by the decree of December 15, 1851.[9] The prefectoral prerogative to issue decrees constituted an accepted and legal exercise of police powers as established by the Revolutionary Law of 12 Messidor An VIII (June 30, 1800), which invested the prefecture of police with the authority to undertake exceptional and repressive measures necessary to protect public order against such threats as epidemics and fires. But in the 1850s, two initiatives—the Law of 1850 and the Napoleonic decrees of 1852 and 1859—had initiated a challenge, hesitantly and somewhat incoherently, to this Revolutionary conception of police powers, by creating new tasks regarding the regulation of insalubriousness as well as placing some old ones under the auspices of an invigorated prefecture of the Seine. Such actions, as we have seen, facilitated a rivalry between the two prefectures that would manifest itself around the definition of insalubriousness as the linchpin of a new, "positive" government of urban life. In the context of this rivalry, which would only escalate under Napoleon's expansive rule (in this regard, the timing of the police decree just after the coup d'état of December 2, 1851, was hardly coincidental), the 1851 decree did not simply aim at applying existing laws to the problem of disease. Rather, it sought to transform the quality and extent of the police regulation of disease so as to make it indispensable to a new practice of government in Paris.

Not all of the provisions contained in the decree were new. For example, the neighborhood commissions would assist the police in regulating public instances of insalubriousness, like "hazardous" industries or the illegal dumping of garbage. Within this category, commissions would also assume the task of maintaining public morality in their neighborhoods, an objective that had been connected to the "policing" of public insalubriousness since at least the middle of the eighteenth century. In 1862, M. Fuilhan, a member of the commission in the fifteenth arrondissement, called attention to the presence of prostitutes on the rue de l'École. "Girls of the worst sort," he reported, "inhabit the ground floor opening onto the public way, observing no law, accosting the passersby in plain daylight and devoting themselves to public acts of obscenity, which makes the way of the street impossible for honest women."[10] Complaints about prostitutes hanging out of the windows of certain dwellings on the rue François Miron were often discussed at the weekly meetings of the fourth arrondissement Commission. And again, in the recently created fifteenth arrondissement, another commission member, M. Gendron, pointed out the harm to the public health resulting from water left stagnating in the pits of the fortifications; what is more, he argued, public morals are offended by the presence of bathers in these passages.[11] Many times, however, the contributions of the commissions to the policing of instances of insalubriousness in public spaces took the form of more mundane discoveries: a broken stair, a sidewalk in need of repair, or the presence on the place des Vosges of vagabonds harassing passersby.

The 1851 decree also made the neighborhood commissions responsible for implementing regulatory measures on a local level in the event of an epidemic crisis. Here, the decree institutionalized on a permanent basis those tasks that the ephemeral commissions d'hygiène and the bureaux de bienfaisance had carried out on a temporary and ad hoc basis during the cholera crises of 1832 and 1849. Like their predecessors, the new commissions would deliver *secours* (medications, blankets, and financial support), offer *conseils* (instructions for the prevention of cholera), and perform home checks (to discover and treat the early symptoms of cholera as well as to inform the prefect of "causes of insalubriousness" that produced disease). But the prefect of police used the permanent establishment of these commissions to replace the traditional emphasis on delivering assistance (*secours*), usually supplied by the bureaux de bienfaisance during epidemic crises, with the search for causes of insalubriousness in private dwellings. Now the activity of the bureaux would be subordinated to the control of the commissions during times of epidemic crises and, along with it, the role of "assistance" to a preventive regulation focused on identifying and regulating the causes of insalubriousness in the home. During the cholera scare of 1853, M. Trébuchet, chief of the Bureau de la salubrité at the prefecture of police, informed the commission of the fifth arrondissement that "the organization of assistance will be the same as in 1849; one has only suppressed the [former] neighborhood commissions to allow the *bureaux de secours*, under the exclusive direction of the *commissions d'hygiène et de salubrité d'arrondissement*." He proceeded to complete his instructions by focusing exclusively on the search for "causes of insalubriousness in homes."[12]

This emphasis on regulating the home during epidemic crises held out important and novel political implications, containing the seeds of change in the character of urban government. By marginalizing assistance, the prefecture of police rejected a mode of government centered around intermittent provisioning of the poor and floating population of Paris. The new focus on the home posited, in its place, a politics of integration that made "residence" the sine qua non for governing a rapidly changing urban population. The mayor and chief of the fourth arrondissement commission expressed his dissatisfaction with assistance as a mode of government: "Everyone demands and would even demand more while the bureau which demands nothing from anyone does not have enough funds to assist all the poor and sick without distinctions."[13] While the prefect of police had always considered the exceptional regulation of the home as part of his general task to protect the safety and the security of the population, the decree regularized and institutionalized the search for causes of disease in the home. It did so by linking the causes of disease to the demographic changes of an urbanizing and industrializing city, in the process making necessary a more consistent and invasive regulation of domestic space. In an 1878 circular, the prefect informed the commissions of their responsibility and authority to regulate the danger to public health posed by the city's *"population flottante,"* dangers that (in the context of this circular) would be exacerbated by the upcoming Universal Exposition:

> So, to summarize, the activity of police can be exercised in both private and public space for everything that concerns health. It is a question here of a compelling interest before which all private interest must bow. Also, the powers invested in municipal authority for preventing or repressing dangers are most extensive. . . ."[14]

The political implications of the central position assigned to regulating the insalubrious home in the Decree of 1851 went beyond simply finding new ways of integrating a "floating population" into the structures of urban life. More important, at issue here was who would define and regulate the problem of the insalubrious home as the center of a new practice of urban government. For the Law of 1850 had envisioned a new regulation of the home that largely excluded policing. And, so it seems, the Prefectoral Decree of 1851 responded by attempting to "recapture" the insalubrious home as an object of police regulation. That intent was more clearly pronounced in the third major provision of the decree, which instructed the commissions to assist the Commission on Insalubrious Dwellings in searching out insalubrious dwellings. Here, in an ironic twist, the neighborhood commissions that existed under the auspices of the prefect of police would help the prefect of the Seine to implement a law that had been intended, in part, to restrict the authority of the prefecture of police but that had failed to specify an effective mechanism by which municipalities could "discover" insalubrious homes (the law simply empowered them to act on complaints filed by tenants). The prefectoral decree would supplement an inadequate law by directing the neighborhood commissions to inform the Commission on Insalubrious Dwellings of their discovery of suspect dwellings. The secretary general of the neighborhood hygiene commissions explained this to the fourth arrondissement commission in 1859:

> The only power that the law places at the disposition of the [police] administration to intervene regards boardinghouses [and not workers' apartments]; however, it is reassuring to recognize that if there is a lapse in the present [1850] legislation in this matter, the [neighborhood] commission knows how to supplement it and its conciliatory intervention leads to impressive results.[15]

It would be hard to deny that the prefecture of police offered the neighborhood commission's assistance here as a way of extending its own regulation of the insalubrious home, that ill-defined and contested space where the future shape of urban government would be forged. In this matter, the prefecture's trump card was *exécution d'office*: It possessed the power to discover, prescribe, and enforce regulations regarding insalubriousness that had been denied to the prefecture of Seine and that had limited the ability of the latter to fulfill the duties enumerated in the 1850 law. In the end, the role of the neighborhood commissions to assist the on Insalubrious Dwellings only fueled the acrimonious competition between the two prefectures.

The minutes of the commissions in four very different arrondissements—the first, fourth, fifth, and fifteenth—all exhibit a consistent and vigorous activity following the 1851 decree, the lengthy lapses following the 1871 Paris Commune uprising notwithstanding.[16] To be sure, the problems pursued by each commission varied according to the character of the arrondissement. The fifteenth arrondissement, for example, incorporated into the city limits only in 1860, was more sparsely populated than the first or fifth; its commission was more preoccupied with the industries sprouting up there after Haussmann's demolitions had exiled (at least some of them) from the "center city." The commission of the fourth arrondissement, which included much of the Marais, was more concerned with the long-standing problem of unhealthful dwellings that Haussmann's selective rebuilding in the center city had only exacerbated. In the fifth arrondissement, home to a very poor population, the Bureau de bienfaisance maintained a more vigorous activity than elsewhere.[17]

Despite these differences, however, all commissions confronted the pressing question concerning the substance and extent of their authority to enter the home as stipulated in the 1851 decree. That decree had instructed the commissions to assist the prefects in regulating insalubriousness, especially where the "silence of the law" (such as the 1850 Law on Insalubrious Dwellings) provided inadequate regulatory provisions. But the commissions were invested with no legal power to enter homes or enforce their findings of insalubriousness, except perhaps in certain urgent circumstances such as epidemics, where commission members became authorized as agents of the prefecture of police who could compel property owners to remove potential causes of insalubriousness (even this conferral of power was questionable). In calmer times, commission members acted "officiously"; they pursued an *"intervention amiable,"* encouraging residents to allow them access to houses or to undertake improvements. This officious activity was premised upon the limited capacities of government to intervene in social life; it aimed at convincing the individual of the necessity to act where government was not empowered to do so. While lacking the coercive power of an official legislative mandate, an officious intervention was potentially effective precisely because it could gain entrance to a home where the law, bound up with the right of property, could not. By relying upon the officious interventions of neighborhood commissions, the prefecture of police could also avoid the cumbersome mechanisms sometimes necessitated by the rule of law (like judicial review of regulatory activities). Thus, in an 1859 letter sent to the prefect of police, the fourth arrondissement commission celebrated the efficacy of its intervention:

> We know that officially we must conform to article six of the decree of 15 December 1851—but if we only acted officially what would we do? What would we accomplish? Mostly nothing, while by the officious approach we spare the administration considerable work which it would not be able to execute very rapidly . . . and which the local commission realizes with such instruments that spare its subjects from inconveniences.[18]

But almost immediately after the establishment of the commissions, questions arose about what it meant for a commission member to act "officiously." Moreover, because commission members acted on behalf of the prefecture of police, these questions highlighted the politically charged problem of the regulation of insalubriousness in the capital. The first question addressed whether, during an epidemic crisis, the commissions could enter the home to discover causes of insalubriousness and order their suppression. In 1853, when the threat of cholera seemed "imminent," the fourth arrondissement commission communicated to the prefect its confusion regarding the "*recherche à domicile des causes d'insalubrité*":

> These instructions have been interpreted differently by a member of a section composed of zealous and devoted men; [he] insists on visiting one by one the houses in his district. To accomplish his mission fully according to his wishes, the member thought to have the right even to enter into the interior of the residence. On this last point, the other two sections . . . held different opinions.[19]

Here, two problems arose. How did the prefect of police confer an "official" authority on the commissions to enter the home during times of epidemic crisis? Could the prefecture of police delegate its authority? Commissions were constantly requesting from the prefect palpable signs of authority that they could present to landlords: calling cards, medals, and posters attesting to the official status of neighborhood commission members. At the April 1872 meeting of the fifth arrondissement commission, only the second since the Commune had disrupted its activities, M. Michan expressed "the fear that the commission remains powerless before the ill will [of landlords and concierges] and asks if any coercive means exist, if the decisions of the commission will carry a sanction."[20] The prefect often replied not with bronze, but with the authority of official judicial pronouncements, like the circular written in 1878, in which he stated that "[t]he Cour de cassation recognized on March 24, 1866, that municipal officers always have the right to enter the dwellings of citizens during the day for specific reasons determined by law, and notably for all questions concerning police, public health and security, as conferred by the law to their vigilance."[21] But such misleading pronouncements—misleading because they failed to address whether a commission member was a municipal officer or whether the particular scenario of the commission could be considered as an *"objet spécialement déter-miné par la loi"*—only revealed the contested nature of police author-ity to enter the home and so did little to assuage the uneasiness of commissions in their attempted interventions.

These problems arose only when cholera seemed imminent—1853, 1865, 1873. But house checks also occupied the commissions on a daily basis, as the Decree of 1851 instructed them to assist the Commission on Insalubrious Dwellings in finding unhealthful dwellings. Here problems of a different sort arose. Did their officious capacity in this regard enable commission members to suggest repairs to landlords? And if not, which prefect should receive their reports on homes? Should they send the reports to the prefect of the Seine, who admin-istered the Commission on Insalubrious Dwellings? Or should they send reports directly to the authority responsible for the administra-tion of the neighborhood commissions—the prefecture of police? Once again, the four arrondissements analyzed here bear witness to numerous and contradictory interpretations. M. DuPuy of the fif-teenth arrondissement recommended

> to the commission to abstain from making absolute prescriptions re-garding work to be executed by property owners in matters of health. The preferred [procedure] will be to verify the problem, inform the authorities, and indicate the remedies or modifications to bring to the state of things. But it is necessary to refrain from conciliatory advice which would perhaps lead property owners to commit infractions with-out their knowing it, and which would involve the responsibility of the Commission d'arrondissement. Legal prescriptions are the job of the Commission des logements insalubres, and it's up to the prefecture of the Seine to initiate legal proceedings.[22]

But just a few months before DuPuy's cautious advice to his commis-sion—which discouraged his fellow members from even making sug-gestions on an officious basis—the mayor of the fourth arrondisse-ment encouraged a wider activity for his commission: "The Mayor engaged the members to invite, as they have always done in the past, property owners to visit their buildings and execute the necessary re-pairs."[23] Twelve years later, in 1872, the president of that same com-mission (who was probably also the mayor of the arrondissement) articulated a more modest vision of its activity. "The mission of the commission," he said, "is confined to formulating suggestions, which are sent to the appropriate authority, who will pursue them."[24]

Even the secretary general of the commissions, appointed by the prefect of police to attend the meetings of the various commissions and to monitor their activities, provided the commissions with conflicting interpretations about the extent of their responsibility regarding home checks. In 1868, M. Poisson entered the not infrequent debate over the fourth arrondissement commission's responsibilities by "attributing" to it "a role of simple verification."[25] At the December 1872 meeting of the fifth arrondissement, his successor, M. Hébrard, expanded upon Poisson's somewhat modest vision: "[O]ne reminds the commission members that their competence and intervention can be usefully extended beyond the limits strictly defined by the printed instructions that the prefecture puts at their disposal."[26]

This confusion over commission attributions exacerbated the rivalry between the two prefectures. The prefecture of the Seine was content to allow the commissions to verify the presence of unhealthful dwellings—after all, the Law of 1850 did not invest it with statutory power to search out dwellings. While accepting the assistance of the neighborhood commissions, the prefecture jealously guarded against their going beyond the act of verifying the existence of insalubrious dwellings [*constatation*]. In 1860, the prefect of the Seine wrote to the fifth arrondissement commission that "the Commission des logements insalubres alone has the right to indicate the sanitary measures to be imposed on property owners." But the prefect did not practice the same respect for prefectoral attributes that he preached. He requested from the first arrondissement that it send reports of insalubrious dwellings directly to him, as opposed to the past practice of transmitting them indirectly through the prefect of police. The mayor of the first arrondissement was all too willing to point out that trespass to his superior, the prefect of the Seine: "[I] permit myself, Mr. Prefect, to inform you that this request contradicts the instructions of the Prefect of Police which accompanied the decree of 15 December 1851 and which indicate that it is he alone who must transmit the reports of the hygienic councils [*sic*] when they pertain to questions outside of his competence."[27]

The prefect of police, for his part, was always in search of abuses committed by the prefect of the Seine. In an 1860 letter to the fourth arrondissement, he had criticized the habit of some commissions to "send their reports directly to the Commission des logements insalubres on buildings whose bad condition seems to require the transfer to this commission." He went on to remind this neighborhood commission that the 1852 ordinance specifying the responsibilities of the commissions mandated the transmission of *all* reports to his office.[28] Such homage to regulatory boundaries, however, did not prevent the prefecture of police from attempting to expand the horizon of its jurisdiction. We have already seen the Circular of 1878, which justified the widest possible police regulation of insalubrious homes considered "dangerous" to public health (this ordinance, it should be pointed out, was not issued at a "crisis" moment, such as the imminent threat of cholera, but in the context of an impending Universal Exposition). The president of the fifth arrondissement commission summarized for his colleagues what was probably the same circular: "[T]he legislator wished to invest the municipal authority with the most extensive rights in that which concerns the public health; the members of the commission have an absolute right of surveillance and inspection over public space . . . and even over private dwellings that risks coming up against the principle of the liberty of industry and the inviolability of the home, which must bow before the general interest."[29] While the circular, as presented here, was a gross exaggeration of the regulation of the insalubrious home by police powers, it indicates why commissions might have expressed bewilderment at the aggressive and contradictory pronouncements concerning the authority of the respective prefectures.

What needs to be avoided here is an instrumentalist interpretation that frames prefectoral ambition as the reason for the confusion over the commission's role and its officious authority. The problems that commissions encountered were not the result of two competitive prefects who distorted the transparent letter of the law for the benefit of their own power. Rather, the rivalry and contradictory interpretations themselves resulted from the two ill-conceived regulatory realms of insalubriousness that were at the center of the mid-century effort to transform the conception and practice of urban government. The Law of 1850 adopted the insalubrious home to distinguish the regulatory spheres of an increasingly restricted prefecture of police and an expanding prefecture of the Seine. But the principles that defined those spheres were neither complementary nor comparable, thus leading to regulatory confusion. The law did restrict the authority of police over the insalubrious home by making the prefecture of the Seine responsible for encouraging landlords to remove permanent causes of insalubriousness. The law, however, did not eliminate the police regulation of the "danger" posed by the insalubrious home as the source of epidemic disease; thus, the police power to regulate epidemic disease remained intact. It was unclear, however, when the problem of permanent causes of insalubriousness in dwellings became a danger subject to police powers. Did the imminence of cholera return the home to police regulation? The neighborhood commissions reproduced the confusion of prefectoral responsibilities and jurisdictions with interventions characterized alternately by modesty and excess. Either they were reluctant to implement the police power to enter the home—even during times of epidemic disease—or they went beyond the simple task of verifying the presence of insalubrious homes by suggesting and enforcing repairs. In the end, such ambivalent behavior only reflected a deeper confusion about the regulation of insalubrious dwellings and the vision of urban government that such a regulation was intended to realize.

### III. Scientific Intervention

In 1879, on the eve of the decade that would establish the Republic's definitive victory, the question of commission authority dissipated in a flurry of activity. That activity began with three directives sent by the prefecture of police to the commissions. The first directive was the transmission of a request from the minister of agriculture for statistics on the incidence of contagious disease. (Up until 1879, only statistics on deaths had been collected in Paris under the auspices of the prefecture of the Seine and its *médecins de l'état civil*.) Beginning in 1878, this information was organized into an annual

report on epidemic disease in Paris, under the direction of the Conseil d'hygiène publique. In 1882, the prefecture requested from the
commissions information on the incidence of typhoid fever in their
respective arrondissements as the basis for an *enquête* that it intended to produce on the puzzling etiology of the disease; most
likely, the information was used by Auguste Ollivier for the 1888
*Rapport sur la fièvre typhoïde à Paris et sa prophylaxie*, also published
under the auspices of the conseil.[30] The mayor of the fifth arrondissement informed the commission: "An *enquête* has been initiated on
the pathology of typhoid fever. It is a question of investigating the
telluric, topographical, hygienic conditions, the circumstances of
home, crowding, food, [and] immigration which can facilitate the
development of the disease."[31]

Finally, beginning in 1879 and 1880, the prefecture began to inform the commissions of smallpox cases in their neighborhoods that
had been reported to it by the hospital administration, the Assistance
publique. The role of the commissions was to confirm that a case of
smallpox had occurred at the address indicated by the prefecture of
police and to inform that office of the *"causes d'insalubrité"* in the
dwelling that were deemed responsible for the outbreak. The 1879
annual report of the fifth arrondissement recognized the importance
of this task in the daily work of the commission: "The smallpox epidemic which developed during the first days of this year has been a
stimulant for [commission members]. They hastened to visit the
homes where death by smallpox had been pointed out to them, and
they have prescribed everywhere preventive measures."[32]

By 1886, these checks had been extended to all contagious diseases, with the exception of tuberculosis, that afflicted the capital.
These visits invigorated the commissions to such an extent that an
annual report of their activity—hitherto published by the prefecture
of police only intermittently and unenthusiastically—began to appear
regularly. In the report for the year 1884, Martellière, the guiding
force behind the active commission of the second arrondissement,
considered the examination of homes in which contagious disease
had supposedly occurred as the focal point of his commission's work.
"In recent years," he wrote, "the vast majority of these visits, which

had already greatly increased, took place on the demand of the administration in the event of a case of epidemic disease, smallpox and typhoid fever."[33] The prefecture of police would more forcefully assert its control over these investigations in 1884 through the establishment of the Bureau des épidémies, reorganized in 1892 as the Service des épidémies; henceforth, the commissions would be responsible mainly for the investigation of *"causes d'insalubrité"* in dwellings where a case of contagious disease had come to the attention of a new prefectoral (bureau) servant—the *médecin délégué*.

It is important to note what is not new here. There was no new law passed or new decree issued that would have transformed the activity of the commissions. Neither did the form of the home check change; commission members, as always, inspected courtyards, stairways, communal toilets (there were few private bathrooms in most of these apartment dwellings), and individual dwellings. What did change was the remaking, in the context of the Pasteurian debates, of the commission intervention into an act of scientific knowledge. According to the 1897 annual report of the conseil:

> An *enquête* on the salubriousness of an apartment house is not a matter, as it was fifty years ago, of a superficial glance; to be serious and complete, it requires a full day; it cannot be accomplished without having at hand *sous les yeux* the plans of the home and subsoil, the (non-drinking) water lines and the toilets, the wells, the garbage dumps, the drinking water mains.[34]

Here, the use of the term *enquête*, the rejection of unreflective observation (*"simple coup d'oeil"*) in favor of a critical expertise (*"sous les yeux les plans de la maison"*), connotes a new perception of the scientific aims and rigor of commission house checks. Moreover, the commissions undertook an *enquête* not as a discrete, intermittent scientific exercise, but rather made it into an ongoing process that formed the basis for a permanent regulation of contagious disease. "No one doubts," wrote a member of the first arrondissement commission,

> the immense importance of a thorough and serious *enquête* on each building in the arrondissements. Each house then would have its own health record (*casier de salubrité*) on which one could record the cases of

contagious disease that might develop there. The record, in the event of an epidemic, would have the advantage of permitting authorities to know in advance the weak and menacing points and to act accordingly.

During the 1884 epidemic, the tenth arrondissement did just that, increasing its membership to ninety in order to check the salubriousness of all its dwellings (thirty-five hundred in all); these visits established a permanent record of the arrondissement, especially relating to its history of and potential for disease.

The scientific value of the commission intervention developed in the context of the debate over the etiology of contagious diseases. It is significant that Lagneau, a member of the conseil who edited the annual commission report during the first years of its publication, praised the scientific competence of the commissions from the lectern of the Academy of Medicine during the 1882 session. "The hygienic commissions," he waxed, "know perfectly the causes of insalubriousness in their neighborhoods."[35] By 1882 the academy was embroiled in a debate over the sufficiency of the microbe as the basis for explaining contagious disease (typhoid fever was the central preoccupation of academy members during this year), and hygienists like Brouardel and Arnould (soon to be followed by Kelsch) had begun to reformulate, from a social viewpoint, its status as the cause of disease. As we have seen, this debate was concerned largely with certain puzzles of transmission—why some people exposed to infection could resist the development of pathological symptoms, why a generalized source of infection (like a water supply) resulted in sporadic clusters of disease, why these clusters reappeared periodically despite new sources of infection—that could not be explained in terms of Pasteur's exteriorized microbe. Because these puzzles suggested the centrality of local, social influences, the home check became highly regarded as a source of scientific knowledge in the highest echelons of late-nineteenth-century French scientific inquiry.

The officious local intervention of commission members produced useful information inaccessible to the experimental method. They confirmed the reality of the cases that were reported to the prefect by the hospital administration (Assistance publique), the only available source for morbidity statistics before the obligatory declaration provision of the 1892 law on the regulation of the medical profession. The information that administration provided was not always reliable, given the reluctance of Parisians, who hated the hospitals and only used them when absolutely necessary, to offer accurate information on their civil status. But these statistics supplied the necessary preliminary information upon which an explanation and regulation of contagious disease could be based. Commissions confirmed and complemented this information. They used their familiarity with the geography and population of their arrondissements to place seemingly isolated reported cases of disease in larger patterns of contagion. They were especially skillful in obtaining information about water supply, the conditions of toilets in apartment houses, and the habits of immigrants that would help in understanding latency and other complex, indirect mechanisms of contagion. In 1895, M. Marcelin of the first arrondissement visited an apartment on the rue du Pont Neuf, no. 22. His visit made him recall "that about three months ago, a case of scarlet fever broke out, and the disinfection was performed only after two other cases recently appeared. He stated this troubling coincidence."[36]

Here, the sharp memory of a zealous commission member recast this isolated case of scarlet fever as a product of contagion that could now be explained by the insalubrious conditions of the apartment building. An equally devoted and perceptive member of the fifteenth arrondissement discovered that an infant residing on rue Lecourbe had been the origin of an isolated outbreak of smallpox—an *"épidémie de maison"*—by noting the "coincidence" of five cases in surrounding buildings, as well as one case at a dwelling on the nearby rue Vanneau, which the infant had visited each day. In the member's report (we don't know his name), he admitted the probable existence of other cases that escaped his attention and that would remain unknown, in the process emphasizing the centrality of his local expertise in resolving the scientific conundrum of transmission.

Through such efforts, the commissions contributed to shaping the *foyer* as a category of scientific explanation of contagious disease. The term had been used as early as the cholera epidemic of 1832 as a way of specifying the location of disease.[37] But beginning in the 1880s, hygienists began to employ it to define local conditions, and especially the conditions of the home, as the force behind the revival of disease that explained irregular patterns of contagion or contagion without "importation." By doing so, the commissions helped to unify the two sides of the debate about contagious disease that had come to be fractured in the role of the germ versus the role of the terrain. The category of the *foyer* developed the scientific authority of the commissions in other ways. For the *foyer* was prescriptive as well as explanatory. It articulated a method of combating contagious disease that made local knowledge an act of prevention. If the revival of latent germs caused epidemic outbreaks, and if that revival could be traced to banal conditions of insalubriousness in the home, then an effective regulatory system had to search out those conditions and prevent them from serving as the origin of an epidemic outbreak. This prophylactic goal would be realized through two acts: (1) to find and control the sporadic cases of contagious disease before they became generalized and (2) to ensure salubrious conditions throughout the city as a barrier against these ever present, ever menacing sporadic cases. Here, we are reminded of the regulatory vision articulated by Dujardin-Beaumetz, the first director of the Service des épidémies: "Preventive hygiene is not possible if one does not know the first cases of an epidemic that one must fight; it is imperative to extinguish these first cases in their *foyer*, whence the necessity of knowing them."[38]

The centrality of the commission intervention in articulating and regulating the *foyer* served as the point of departure for the extension of police authority over the home. Once hygienists and commission members had defined the conditions of the insalubrious home as the basis for the scientific understanding of contagious disease in urban life, the home became redefined as a danger subject to constant police regulation. According to the 1888 report of the nineteenth arrondissement, "The building inhabited in common needs a serious surveillance which, if it is not prescribed by law, is well indicated in the public administration regulations. Besides, there are always epidemics in Paris. The prefect [of police] can always be the master in these cases of public health."[39] The perception and regulation of the dangerous home were dependent upon the "local" expertise of commission members, their ability to access and interpret a whole gamut of information about the dwelling that "identified" its status as a *foyer*. Where their officious capacity had once expressed the limitations of government intervention, the commissions' newly constituted scientific authority now vastly expanded the possibilities of police intervention in the contested space of the dwelling.

When the eleventh arrondissement trio of Motet, Pontier, and Signez professed in their 1891 report that "to foresee the illness is to combat it,"[40] they were not only affirming the importance of prevention (*prévoir*) as the basis of a regulatory system, but also defining the hygienic act of "seeing" (*voir*) the local conditions of disease as integral to a preventive system of regulation. An 1887 report by the same commission affirmed more explicitly the centrality of a uniquely "hygienic" expertise to an expanded policing of disease: "There are none among us who could not designate beforehand in our respective neighborhoods the points which would be hard hit by a sudden epidemic."[41] The elaboration of the *foyer* through the commission intervention remade the politically contested administrative category of the "insalubrious home" into a scientifically verifiable danger, subject to constant police observation that would be exercised by the expert commissions.

The scientific imperative to know and regulate the danger posed by the insalubrious home emboldened the commissions to perform home checks in a way that administrative pronouncements of its dangers in the past (like the police circular of 1878) had failed to do. The prefect of the Seine noted the increased activity of the commissions and acted to control it. In 1883, he appointed, with the approval of the prefect of police, a member of the Commission on Insalubrious Dwellings to sit on each of the arrondissement commissions as a way of monitoring what he considered

> the habit acquired by some *commissions d'hygiène* of prescribing certain improvements to the owners of insalubrious buildings. It results that the Commission des logements insalubres, called in turn to verify the same buildings, can prescribe completely different improvements from those already executed on the advice of the commission d'hygiène.[42]

But now, acting as a scientific authority, neighborhood commission members began to respond to the territorial claims of the Commission on Insalubrious Dwellings (and through it, to the prefect of the Seine) in a more aggressive manner. Dr. Tissier "affirmed that the Commission d'hygiène of the fourth arrondissement is composed of sufficiently competent members and that the delegate of the Commission des logements insalubres is not qualified to judge the numerous and diverse questions which are submitted to it. In the final analysis, the need to defer to the propositions made by the members of the Commission des logements insalubres will delay the tasks of the Commission [d'hygiène]."[43]

In an attempt to secure its rapidly diminishing jurisdiction over the insalubrious home, the prefecture of the Seine asserted its own scientific capacities by extending the functions of the Municipal Statistical Service, headed by the eminent statistician Jacques Bertillon.[44] While the office was concerned primarily with verifying the deaths in the department and issuing death certificates, it began to collect morbidity statistics in 1880. Throughout the 1880s and 1890s, however, neighborhood commission members pointed out the inadequacies of the Seine's initiative. In his 1892 report on the cholera epidemic in the Paris suburb of St. Denis, commission member Roy des Barres commented on the discrepancy between the statistics gathered by the Service des épidémies (877) and the Statistique municipale (265). Because cholera existed sporadically before assuming an epidemic form, he argued, the early cases were difficult to diagnose and often ended up being categorized as a banal disease with symptoms resembling those associated with cholera—*"diarrhée cholériforme," "cholérine,"* or *"choléra nostras."* In his view, the expert medical inspectors associated with the service, Dubief and Thoinot, were able to diagnose correctly those preliminary cases whose detection was necessary for the successful regulation of epidemic disease. "The *enquêtes* that these two medical inspectors of the Service des épidémies have undertaken for each case during the entire epidemic have permitted them to establish the real cause of death and to furnish to the prefect very precise information that the analysis of death certificates cannot provide with sufficient exactitude."

Roy des Barres indirectly suggested the reason for the disparity in skills and success exhibited by the respective prefects when he stated that the "interest in [performing] investigations immediately is to know the exact extent of the ravages produced by these afflictions." His use of the term "immediate" posed the criticism of the Seine's "verifiers" widely held by commission members: Out of respect for family autonomy, the *médecins de l'état civil* interrogated the family of the deceased only after a "decent" interval (perhaps two days) and then posed their questions delicately so as not to offend the grieving family. But the commissions, acting as agents of science and the police that protected the public from "danger," would not be impeded by the principle of individual liberty or respect for family privacy that had prevented the Statistique municipale from furnishing rapid and detailed information about the crucial early cases of contagious disease. It was the traditional police interest in aggressively investigating a "danger" that allowed the commissions to obtain a "certain" knowledge of contagious disease. For Roy des Barres, the conclusion imposed itself: "[I]t would be desirable to see the director of the Municipal Statistical Service under the auspices of the Conseil d'hygiène publique et de salubrité, which would then be able to have knowledge of the documents gathered by the prefecture of police."[45]

Roy des Barres's report suggests the complex relationship between scientific authority and police authority that emerged during the 1880s. It was not simply that, as Lagneau wrote in 1881, "*la statistique signale le danger.*"[46] Rather, the relationship between policing and science was symbiotic. For in the 1880s, both scientific knowledge about contagious disease and the authority of police were in crisis. While the debates over etiology in the Academy of Medicine had revealed the insufficiency of Pasteur's understanding of the microbe as the basis for understanding and regulating disease, so too the campaign against the police regulation of prostitution and the revival of the municipal council's call for autonomy beginning in the 1870s put into question, in terms more forceful than ever before, the role of policing in Republican urban government. Ultimately, each found "completion" in the other. For, just as the commission's local and officious authority provided the basis for assessing and regulating those local social conditions that explained the sporadic and irregular transmission of contagious disease in Paris, so too the debate over the etiology of contagious disease transformed the commission's officious capacity into a scientific authority that made possible an expanded conception and practice of policing.

The contribution of the first arrondissement commission to the *enquête* on typhoid fever illuminates this symbiotic relationship. In an 1883 report, the commission member Duroziez examined all of the factors that could spread typhoid fever in urban life. Direct contact, air, water: All appeared important but not compelling. The provisional conclusion of his report was not encouraging: "We doubt that the question can be resolved for Paris." Duroziez continued by focusing on the role of immigrants in the transmission of typhoid fever: "In the worst hit neighborhoods, how many provincial immigrants are there?" Here he found that the incessant movement of the immigrant, the lack of a fixed place in the city, rendered it difficult to understand his or her role in the etiology of the disease: "How can we evaluate the population of the neighborhood of Les Halles?" He concluded by advocating the regulation of the insalubrious home as the best defense against contagious disease:

> We can only do what the Conseil and the commissions do, improve the unhealthy dwellings, prevent the crowding of individuals, widen the streets, provide noncontaminated water, call for the construction of affordable housing[;] but whatever is done, the population which pours in from the countryside will always make the Paris dwelling dangerous.

Here, Duroziez's selection of the home as the appropriate answer to the problem of contagious disease became comprehensible because it fulfilled simultaneously three criteria. It gathered in a coherent unity all the various etiological factors—air, overcrowding, water, social habits—that, taken separately, could not provide a compelling explanation of how typhoid fever spread in urban life. Second, it furnished a plausible solution to the problem of immigrants that dominated the middle part of his *enquête*. The focus on the home did not simply reveal the role of immigrants in transmitting typhoid fever. It simultaneously provided a way of knowing and regulating a segment of the population whose movement had always rendered it ungovernable. Third, Duroziez endorsed the regulation of the home, paradoxically, because it was an imperfect solution to the problem of contagious disease in Paris. The home embodies the ever-present potential of disease in urban life. Always dangerous, the home must always be subject to police powers. The interest in extending and transforming police authority as part of a consistent, positive government of urban social life brought coherence to the insalubrious house as the "dangerous" origin of epidemic disease whose "reality" subsequently was invoked to justify the extension of police powers.[47]

## IV. Disease Regulation and the Socialized Individual

At the December 1882 meeting of the fifth arrondissement commission, M. Lecaconnier expressed his reluctance to perform the home checks that the prefect had requested as one of the commission's first scientific interventions: the typhoid fever *enquête*. In Lecaconnier's opinion, the *enquête* required information that would force him to betray the doctor's responsibility to respect the privacy and autonomy of the stricken individual. According to the minutes of that meeting, "he [Lecaconnier] takes refuge behind professional discretion [*le secret professionnel*]." The president of the commission attempted to overcome Lecaconnier's hesitation by arguing that the principle of *secret professionnel* was not applicable in this situation. While it was necessary to gather information about the individual that shed light on the etiology of typhoid fever, such a task constituted an *enquête* on the illness (*maladie*) and not the patient (*malade*).

> One requests from doctors to examine the locations where the disease was declared, to examine the sick person and to investigate the modes of contagion, and to furnish information that they judge useful concerning the etiology of typhoid fever. One does not violate professional discretion by indicating that the illness was preceded by physical exhaustion or moral emotions, since it is not necessary to add what was the reason for physical exhaustion or the source of moral emotions.[48]

By 1897, the commissions had come to understand the complex distinction between *malade* and *maladie*. In November of that year, the first arrondissement commission wrote to the prefect of police that it needed neither the names of individuals nor the exact situation of their dwelling. The only piece of information required was the location of the building; with that minimal indication, the commission would "with all possible discretion establish the character [of the disease], the mode of transmission, the duration of contagion and signal to you the means of preventing its propagation."[49]

The juxtaposition of these two documents displays how the police elaboration of a "scientific intervention" established a conception and practice of social regulation where legislators of the nascent Third Republic could not. It did so by bypassing the juridical field, whose regulatory potential, defined by respect for individual liberty, had left Brouardel with the sterile alternatives of an "authoritarian" law or a "conciliatory" law. Instead, the scientific intervention constituted a new social field through the police investigation and regulation of a danger, the *foyer*. But the latter field could never have been articulated without the former. There could be no *maladie* without a *malade*; the *foyer*, conceived as a danger to society, was intended to resonate in, and transform, another *foyer*, the incubator of the autonomous individual. For the whole problem of contagious disease in nineteenth-century France was bound up with resolving the dilemma that individual liberty posed to the understanding and regulation of social problems. And the *foyer* rearticulated the relationship between the individual and society by revealing them as distinct, though interdependent, entities. In doing so (and this is the reason why the regulation of contagious disease is a crucial chapter in the "making of the Third Republic"),[50] the scientific intervention created within Republicanism a new conception and practice of government as a social force.

Throughout the nineteenth century, the task of regulating contagious disease played on the relationship between individual as *malade* and "individual" as a political construct, the foundational category of post-Revolutionary society. Before the scientific transformations of the 1880s, this relationship was made evident in the home visits undertaken in Paris by the bureaux de bienfaisance and the ephemeral commissions d'hygiène during the cholera crises of 1832, 1849, 1853, and 1865. These "preventive visits" sought out people who displayed the early symptoms of cholera (diarrhea), and provided them with assistance (*"secours"*) for avoiding the development of the full-blown—and usually fatal—stages of the disease. "It is of the utmost importance," the Conseil d'hygiène publique et de salubrité de la Seine advised in its 1853 cholera *Instruction populaire*, "to take care of oneself as soon as a symptom becomes manifest, however slight it is."[51] The "visitors" (they were not all doctors, but notables as well) provided instructions on how the individual should care for him- or herself after the appearance of premonitory symptoms. In an 1832 *Instruction*, E. Moulin, a member of the faculty of the Royal College of St. Louis, wrote that

> [o]ne will make, to much advantage, upon lying down and rising, dry frictions all over the body, to favor perspiration, maintain a soothing warmth and a vital energy. As much as possible, one will avoid exhaustion by work or strenuous activity, late nights, untimely fasting, [and] what would be still more harmful, the excess of the table or women. The abuse of alcohol, drunkenness, in short, could be deadly.[52]

Medications, food, and clothing were offered as well. Most important, financial assistance was given to families where illness, death, or endemic poverty made remunerative work impossible. In 1865, the police commissioner for the suburb of St. Denis informed the prefect of police that he had undertaken home checks to ascertain "the needs of different families in difficult circumstances [*nécessiteux*] in the event that it would become necessary to provide them with assistance."[53]

The medical value of these home checks makes sense within the miasmatic theory of disease that reigned during the first half of the nineteenth century: The individual's best defense against the myriad infections provided by the urban environment was a robust constitution.[54] But the regulation of cholera through the "instruction" and provisioning of cholera victims was also part of a moral education of the "dangerous classes," an attempt to inculcate in them the capacity for individual responsibility and autonomy that defined the possibilities of social order in early-nineteenth-century France.[55] Many of these interventions equated the lack of attention to early symptoms with individual negligence, like the pregnant woman who contracted cholera after attending a friend's wedding celebration or the thirty-nine-year-old Faure Petit Mermet, whose "health failed due to lack of care."[56]

In another example of its moralizing function, Moulin's *Instruction* also aimed at inculcating among the city's poor an aversion for excess, such as those of the "table" and of "women." In this respect, Mermet's death was attributed not only to negligence but excess as well; according to the 1865 police report, "This man, married but without children, works too much." Among the sins of excess, drinking elicited the most severe censure from doctors and commissioners. The fifth arrondissement commissioner reported on a "Sr. Menant": "[His] drunken habits are such that it would be objectionable to provide him with [assistance]. This man has children that it would be proper to place, since he is not worthy of raising them."[57] He would be awarded forty francs only after the children had been removed from the home. This interest in the assumption or abdication of familial roles figured prominently in the delivery of assistance, not simply because it would aid in preventing disease, but because a "properly" constituted home life was viewed as the necessary milieu for the development of a self-regulating individual, the cornerstone of post-Revolutionary society. The prefect of police instructed his commissioners to favor families, and evidence of a respectable family life was often a sufficient criterion for assistance. Thus the mayor of the fifth arrondissement justified the awarding of supplementary assistance by arguing: "M. Patin is a very honest man and a good father [*père de famille*]."[58]

This early-nineteenth-century preventive visit affirmed and nurtured the autonomous subject by caring for the sick person and other family members. The scientific intervention, as institutionalized in the Bureau des épidémies and the service at the end of the century, replaced "caring" with "knowing": The individual came to be regarded as a source of information about a social danger—the *foyer*. In doing so, the scientific intervention minimized the importance of the individual experience of disease and, with it, the "individual." The 1884 enumeration of responsibilities to be assumed by *médecins délégués* (medical delegates), under the direction of the chief medical inspectors at the bureau, captured this transformation in the aims and methods of disease regulation:

> The delegate will not have to concern himself with the individual, the ill person. The ill person will have an attending physician for direct care, or for return to the hospital; [the delegate] will be concerned, above all, with the illness in general, the preservation of the neighbors by all the means that hygiene and experience provide and that the funds allocated by the public authority permit to employ.[59]

Scientific investigation minimized the individual experience of disease in two respects. First, the medical significance of the individual's symptoms was made problematic by the redefinition of disease in terms of cause. Once the focus on the microbial cause had reworked the pathological symptom as the sign, and not the constitutive element, of disease, the individual's symptom became an unreliable tool of diagnosis.[60] Moreover, because microbiological testing was considered unreliable, doctors confirmed the certainty of cholera through simultaneous cases rather than through a deep reading of the individual body. An individual's "abundant" diarrhea and cramps could only suggest cholera; the individual would remain "suspect" until the diarrhea and cramps of other family members or neighbors confirmed contagion. As a result, while the earlier preventive visit had focused on instructing individuals to detect and treat the transparent preliminary stages of cholera, the unreliable status of individual symptoms as "signs" subsequently led the *médecin délégué* to link the intelligibility and concern for the individual experience of disease with those of others. Second, once it was confirmed that the individual suffered from cholera, the objective was to check if the case constituted a *foyer*, that is, whether it could be linked to other simultaneous cases, either as the originator or the consequence of transmission. Once again, therefore, concern for the individual victim became meaningful and necessary only in relation to others.

The bureau initiated an investigation upon receipt of a report that someone had either died or suffered from what appeared to be cholera. This information came from a variety of sources: the Assistance publique, the prefect of the Seine, neighborhood police commissioners, commission members, or even an anonymous letter written by a neighbor. Once reported, the victim became an object of knowledge: a "*cas suspect*." According to Léon Colin,

> Once a suspect case was pointed out to the prefect of police, a nominative white card was filled out and put in alphabetical order, then the inscription of the name and address of the ill person on the sheet. . . . At the same time, a special dossier was opened on the ill person.[61]

The first intervention that followed the creation of the dossier attempted to verify the "suspect" case as a case of contagious disease. Like the "preventive visit," the verification sometimes addressed the symptoms exhibited by the victim. In the 1890 case of a cook named Mme. Masse, Dr. Filibilin wrote: "The death of Madame Masse from cholera seems problematic since I only noted algidity and stomach cramps for symptoms, which one sees in nearly all [cases of] colic and hepatitis."[62] But now doctors interrogated the individual for insight into the nature of the disease. In a report on chicken pox, Auguste Ollivier, a member of the Conseil d'hygiène publique et de salubrité de la Seine, instructed hygienists on the correct procedures for verifying suspect cases: "[I]t is very important to undertake a detailed *enquête* on the subject of the origin of each ill person, one must know not only where he came from, but how he had spent his time during the incubation of the illness."

Unlike the earlier preventive visit, questions about the victim here did not express an interest in aiding or instructing the individual. The *médecin délégué* assumed a blasé attitude—even toward the suffering victim—that reflected the observer-observed relationship of the scientific intervention. In 1890, Dr. Laborderie wrote to the prefect of police: "I was called early yesterday evening to the home of a man named Burgis. . . . He and his wife had taken ill with diarrhea, vomiting, cramps, alas all the symptoms of cholera. The husband will perhaps be dead tonight."[63] That same year, the prefect of police expressed a similarly distanced position toward a M. Granger in a letter to the Assistance publique: "I would be much obliged, Sir, if you would keep me informed about the state of health of the ill person. In the event he should succumb, there would be an interest in performing an autopsy so that the digested materials or the contents of the intestines could be sent to the medical school laboratory." Ironically, the "interest" in the victim as a source of information about a *foyer* makes him more valuable dead than alive.[64]

In interrogating the individual for information about the presence of disease and a potential *foyer*, the *médecin délégué* often interposed himself into relationships that were regarded as the province and expression of the autonomous individual. He promptly questioned the family about the circumstances under which the victim contracted the disease, something the *médecin de l'état civil* was loath to pursue; what is surprising here is to see how often the family cooperated. In the attempt to ascertain whether Albert Reich had died of cholera or food poisoning in 1891, Dujardin-Beaumetz questioned both his wife and the maid about what they had eaten and whether they had experienced any symptoms of illness. The son-in-law of the deceased, who was also a doctor, volunteered to cooperate with Dujardin-Beaumetz's investigation of the circumstances of Reich's death: "I can give you very precise information on the [habits] and on the diverse stages of the disease of M. Reich."[65] The mother of a certain M. Quinquet was more willing to provide information about her son to the authorities than to tend his illness; according to the report, "[t]he mother of M. Quinquet, who did not wish to care for her son [and] with whom she did not live, gave me his vital statistics."[66] In their quest for information, *médecins délégués* did not find it problematic to question the victim's attending physician (*médecin traitant*), and physicians often did not hesitate to respond—even before the 1892 obligatory declaration law.

The interrogation of the individual was not only simultaneously disinterested and intrusive, but brief as well. The verification turned almost immediately to a consideration of others, where the significance of the suspect case—whether or not it constituted a *foyer*—would be found. In an 1885 report to the bureau, the commissioner for the largely proletarian suburb of Aubervilliers compensated for his ignorance of the condition of a mother and daughter, hospitalized with cholera, with a thorough investigation of their family members and neighbors:

As for the family Cotard, 16 rue des Cités, I had no news of the mother and the girl who were brought to the hospital on the 26th. The youngest daughter, whom I had placed in another room, has experienced no symptoms, and it is likely that she will remain immune. The other inhabitants of the contaminated building go about their business. I have not been notified of any new cases in the neighborhood of Quatre Chemins or in the center city.[67]

In 1883, Lagneau was instructed to verify whether the illness of Mme. Henriette Beauvais, seventy-five years old and staying with her daughter during the period of convalescence, was indeed cholera. His report tersely related the symptoms that, in his opinion, signaled cholera: "According to the interns, . . . this ill person experienced strong cramps mainly in the legs, frequent vomiting, liquid feces with yellow lumps." The information provided is both secondhand and impersonal (*"cette malade"*). Lagneau's real concern here was that the prefect had neglected to provide the previous and permanent address of the widow, where she was presumed to have contracted the disease: "I regret that no one gave me the exact address of this ill person, because it would have been wise to ascertain that no other cholera victim was in the neighborhood." The address was subsequently provided, and no other people with similar symptoms had been found; the potential for a *foyer* was avoided.[68] And in the aforementioned case of Albert Reich, Dujardin-Beaumetz supplemented the questioning of the deceased man's wife, maid, and son-in-law/physician with an investigation of the neighborhood in order to confirm the case as cholera or food poisoning. The absence of similar symptoms in the surrounding buildings, coupled with the continued good health of his family members, confirmed food poisoning. (It seems that this *père de famille* ate a great deal more than the others gathered at his table.)

If, as in the case of Albert Reich, the suspect case turned out not to suffer from a contagious disease, the inquiry ended with the verification. If, however, the *médecin délégué* had discovered a case of cholera or typhoid fever, the verification was followed by three preventive measures undertaken by a variety of prefectoral servants: disinfection (prefecture of the Seine), isolation (local police agents), and the identification of *causes d'insalubrité* deemed responsible for the disease (neighborhood hygiene commissions). The same procedures were implemented whether the "case" had resulted in the death or the recovery of the victim. Like the verification before it, the preventive stage of the scientific intervention considered the *malade* only in relation to the interest in the *maladie*: the regulation of the *foyer*.

In the event of a convalescing "case," the *médecin délégué* or commission member attempted to isolate the victim within the existing apartment. The ideal isolation placed the victim in a separate room, with the bed in the middle. But once that objective was realized, the victim became invisible and the intervention turned its attention to those people who surrounded the invalid:

> This question of hygienic precepts, pertaining to individuals who are or must be in contact with choleraics, must be studied from two points of view. It must include the methods one can propose to prevent the individual in contact with the choleraics from contracting cholera and indicate how, by the procedures of disinfection, this person can avoid becoming a *foyer* for propagating the disease.[69]

The 1884 conseil instructions for diphtheria indicated the efforts lavished on regulating the family members whose contact with an invalid could produce a *foyer*:

> 1. It is indispensable to remove any person not involved in the treatment of the ill person, especially children.
> 2. The people who take care of the ill person will avoid kissing him, breathing his exhalations, and placing oneself in front of his mouth during his coughing fits.
> 3. If these people have crevices or small sores either on the hands or face, they will have to cover them with collodion.
> 4. They will eat well, and will have to go out many times during the day for a walk in the fresh air. They will be careful to wash first the face with water containing, per liter, ten grams of boric acid and one gram of thymic acid.
> 5. Finally, they will avoid spending night and day in the room of the sick person.[70]

These instructions were largely reproduced for other diseases as well, with the exception of typhoid fever and cholera instructions, which emphasized the importance of disinfecting excrement believed to carry the germ of both diseases. Measures such as these did not only aim at protecting family members. In 1902, the fifteenth arrondissement undertook an investigation of an "elderly bedridden woman" (no specific disease is given here). According to the report, "[f]eces remained in front of her yarn and on the floor, and the urine infiltrated into the floorboard. All around the bed, the wallpaper is stained, as are the walls, the toilets are dirty. Very unhealthy situation for the residents [of the building] and the neighbors."[71]

In the event of a case resulting in death, the scientific intervention was concerned more with disinfection than with isolation. The real difference, however, resided in the changed attitude toward the family of the victim. While the *médecin délégué* or commission member attempted to prevent the family from becoming a *foyer* through its contact with the convalescent, the family itself was indicted as the potential perpetrator of the *foyer* once the victim had died. In the 1883 report of the second arrondissement, Martellière complained about a family who kept the body of a "young woman" for thirty-six hours after her death from cholera in a cramped apartment whose windows opened onto a narrow street.[72] The 1897 report of the conseil noted "unfortunately" the reluctance of some families, motivated by a "definite modesty" to give their "very dirty and used sheets" to the municipal disinfection service.[73] Perhaps the most frequent complaint lodged against families was their attempt to perform a disinfection without the assistance of an expert commission member or *médecin délégué*. In 1890, M. Lecaconnier, who by now no longer approached an intervention with hesitation, complained about the disinfections that he had evaluated for the bureau: "As for the disinfection of the contaminated location, it was completed superficially; the parents were content to scatter on the floor of the room a carbolic acid solution."[74]

These complaints are interesting because they appear to place the two *foyers* in opposition as a way of removing the obstacle posed by the "inviolable" family to the regulation of disease. The family is implicated in the spread of contagious disease; respect for its integrity and autonomy place society in danger. The reports of the commission

members and *médecins délégués* indicate two ways in which family behavior contributed to the creation of new *foyers* of disease. First, the
individual autonomy and responsibility that the "inviolable" family in
theory is supposed to nurture and that are necessary for preventing
the formation of *foyers* did not exist in practice. Thus, Martellière observed that immigrants did not know the remedy for an infected toilet
and that people in general were "indifferent to the habits of cleanliness," while Rives, a member of the thirteenth arrondissement commission, complained that "families neglected to have a physician
summoned" to treat their children for scarlet fever or mumps.[75] The
1897 conseil report captured the failings of the family in more general
terms:

> It is always necessary to count on the inevitable underhandedness, and if
> not that, the ignorance and negligence of families and persons who care
> for a contagious person. It is the duty of the doctor to point out the
> dangers to the entourage of the patient.[76]

The conclusion was clear: Where the family abdicated its role in preventing the spread of disease, the medical expert would have to intervene. But, second, it is precisely those valorized familial practices and
norms that were seen as facilitating, in certain cases, the transmission
of disease. The "caring" of a wife for her stricken husband, the resistance of a grieving family to get rid of a dead body, the "shame"
[*pudeur*] that prevents certain families from presenting their sullied
garments and bedding to the municipal disinfection service, demonstrated to commission members how familial bonds and values could
produce a deadly *foyer*.

But in the end, the use of individual attributes like *insouciance, ignorance, mauvais vouloir*, or *pudeur* to implicate family members in the
spread of disease suggests a more complex phenomenon than the
simple rejection of the values associated with the autonomous individual or the inviolable family. Rather, these hygienic interventions
rearticulated the category of individualism by making its exercise
conditional upon the recognition of a social interest. The danger embodied in the *foyer* made the acceptance of social duties, articulated
and presented by a regulatory authority, an integral part of what it

means to be an individual in urban space. Thus, when the fifteenth arrondissement commission asked what pressure its members could apply "to persuade a tenant of the interest involved in having the disinfection performed by the [municipal] service and in not leaving it to the care of careless and inexpert tenants," the police commissioner replied that "the [municipal] service which presents itself for disinfection should depend on the methods of persuasion and, without intimidation, exercise a subtle pressure by invoking the general interest."[77]

The scientific intervention of commission members and *médecins délégués* did not only articulate a socialized understanding of individualism that made the enjoyment of freedom dependent upon assuming what government defined as duties toward others, but in negative terms as well: The *foyer* embodied the constant danger that social life posed to the individual. The socialized individual both recognized duties to society and sought protection from the dangers that the threat of disease imposed. In the 1889 report of the second arrondissement commission, Martellière wrote: "The complainant, with a very accurate intuition of the role of the *commissions d'hygiène*, said: 'My neighbors have smallpox, tell me how I can protect myself from them.'"[78] Sometimes the complaints concerned "real" cases of contagious disease or general cases of insalubriousness; other times, it appears renters used the complaint to negotiate, and gain control over, their social environment. Upon investigating a complaint presented by a tenant, the fifteenth arrondissement commission concluded that "[t]he complaint, which emanated from an evicted tenant, seems to be the work of a petty revenge, because the house is well maintained and clean."[79] "Suspect" tenants of buildings—and suspect not simply from the viewpoint of disease—were often the object of these neighborly concerns. Consider this complaint sent anonymously by a landlord to the mayor of the fifth arrondissement in April 1903:

> I have in my house on the rue Maitre Albert, 4, a sick tenant, he is all alone, the other tenants on the landing where he lives have complained for many days, emphasizing the disgusting and sickly odor emitted from his room and person, the concierge of my house has already complained

to the police commissioner to find out what means can be employed to have him removed from the house, he told her it was necessary to bring the complaints of the tenants to the mayor in order to have him removed, for this infection can pose a danger for the tenants.[80]

Whether the *"locataire malade"* was sick or whether the reference to sickness conjured a variety of threats imagined to be posed by this neighbor—or both—is not important here. The letter is illuminating because it reveals that the scientific intervention around the problem of the *foyer* has transformed the popular perception of "inviolable" private space into a social space full of dangers. Moreover, it secured the regulation of this space by creating an ally: the "individual" whose sense of self is expressed and protected through a negotiation with and suspicion of "others." Where the regulatory aspirations of a July Monarchy hygienist like Villermé had foundered upon the principles of individual liberty and the inviolable home, the late-nineteenth-century hygienist successfully rearticulated the relationship between the exercise of individual liberty and the government protection of a larger social interest.

# Conclusion

BY WORLD WAR I, the neighborhood hygiene commissions were largely defunct. As in so many other aspects of the social, political, and economic life of France, the war mobilization and subsequent carnage significantly reduced these efforts, among others, in behalf of regulating disease. The war necessitated a shift in focus, both of resources and interests, from civil life to military life. It facilitated a "demedicalization of the civil milieu,"[1] which rendered French society ill equipped to continue long-standing initiatives such as the campaign against insalubrious housing and tuberculosis or to fight new dangers such as the influenza epidemic of 1918, which killed soldier and civilian with equal ferocity. But the very imperatives of mobilization that had so limited the regulation of disease during World War I ended up reconfirming its crucial role in an enhanced vision of government intervention after the 1918 Armistice.[2] For the war not only made necessary the state assumption of social and economic functions that in peacetime would come to be viewed as a regular facet of government. It also facilitated the political and social integration of a once militant labor movement that henceforth would assume rather than reject the constituted authority of the state.[3] The regulation of disease occupied a conspicuous position in the realization of this expanded vision of the French state. In Paris, neighborhood dispensaries made possible by the 1916 law now proliferated, assuming many of the functions once assigned to the neighborhood hygiene commissions. The ministry of hygiene, assistance, and prévoyance sociale (social welfare) was established in 1920, and state medical functionaries were created in 1941. Health issues were central to the development of the social security system that predominated in the agendas of the Fourth and Fifth Republics after World War II.[4]

These twentieth-century initiatives were so successful, and their identification with Republicanism so seamless, that it is difficult to appreciate the conflict between the Republican principles of individual liberty and the interests of social order that had originally defined the prominent position of disease in nineteenth-century debates about social regulation. That conflict was painfully manifested in the emergence of social suffering and working-class protest that accompanied the advent of industrial society in the 1820s and 1830s. The attempt of the workers' movement to seek an official redress of social suffering—the recognition of "social rights"—sounded a sort of death knell for Enlightenment and Revolutionary understandings of liberty. It did so by revealing that the exercise of political rights would not lead to social harmony—indeed, that political liberty could even produce social disorder. In turn, the provisional Republican government in 1848 responded to the workers' movement with repressive, violent measures that made a mockery of Condorcet's vision of the role of government in shaping the rational self-regulating potential of free individuals.[5] The prominent position of contagion in nineteenth-century social regulation needs to be seen as an attempt to resolve this conflict between liberty and social order by reconstituting them as distinct experiences. Contagion became the obligatory reference point for observing and understanding the myriad problems of industrial society—population growth, overcrowding, poverty, militancy, and disease. As such, it defined social life and social relations in terms of danger, in the process creating "the social" as an object of state regulation.

How contagion effected such a transformation of Republicanism "from within" is best understood by taking into consideration the discursive operations of the human sciences. As a practice that linked knowledge about the individual to the possibilities of state power, the human sciences were grounded in, and invoked, a fractured and highly ambiguous definition of reason. Thus scientists associated with state academies and regulatory bodies referred, in ways both implicit and explicit, to "reason" as the common and human source of knowledge, freedom, and morality in order to define their endeavors (and the relationship between science and the state more generally) as consistent with the institutions and ends of a free society. Yet the very objective and result of their efforts was to remove the possibility of morality from the rational functions of human knowledge and liberty, in the process making the state—and not a conception of the self-regulating individual—the basis for social order.

Such an ambiguous conception of rationality that established the relationship between the human sciences and state power promised to open up a realm of government intervention in social life normally considered to be the sacrosanct sphere of individual autonomy. But the ambiguities inherent in such a fractured conception of scientific rationality sometimes impeded these regulatory efforts, as (I hope) the arduous, century-long preoccupation with the problem of contagion related in this book demonstrates. Hygienists, government regulators, and politicians who were committed to political and economic liberty yet aware of its limited capacity to produce social order nevertheless found it difficult to conceive of liberty and sociability as distinct and (sometimes) oppositional facets of human experience. Many of them could not separate the promise of science from the goal of realizing the free and self-regulating capacities that should define individuals. It was this ambiguous association between scientific rationality, the shaping of individual liberty, and government in a free social order, rather than imperfect scientific techniques or contradictory evidence, that explains the debates between Villermé and Buret, or between Brouardel and Arnould, concerning the causes of contagious disease and their implications for the government regulation of social life. The character of that association also explains the commitment of Republican politicians to producing a legal regulation of contagious disease, as well as their incapacity or unwillingness to confront the limited potential of law to legitimize such a profound government intervention in social life, and especially in the home.

In the end, however, these efforts to redefine, through contagion, social order as a task of government yielded impressive and highly original, if sometimes unexpected, results. They produced a diverse, energetic, and often contentious field of scientific inquiry about disease. And they ended up creating, through the scientific investigation and regulation of disease, a vastly transformed conception and practice of policing as the basis for a prescriptive, moral government in a Republican social order. The originality of some of these results surprised contemporary observers and participants themselves, and many were reluctant to acknowledge them as evidence for the triumph of Republicanism at the end of the nineteenth century. For the very same reason, these regulatory endeavors have also escaped the attention of historians who, by taking for granted a definition of the free individual as moral and self-regulating, of scientific truth as linked to the realization of this conception of the rational self-regulating individual, and of "law" as their preferred and common instrument, have failed to grasp the complexity of science as a discursive field that reconfigured the relationship between the individual, social order, and government regulation. Behind the performative statements of Third Republic legislators who claimed that attention to the problem of disease would ultimately realize the Republican promise of individual liberty as the basis of social order, or hygienists who claimed to pursue an explanation and regulation of disease untainted by political interests, there exist complex and important connections between science and the attempt to extend the role of government in a free social order. It is here that a history of Republicanism, and how it confronted and ultimately surpassed the contradictions and limitations of individual liberty revealed by the problems of poverty and working-class militancy in industrial society, needs to begin.

Even in twentieth-century France, where the incorporation of a once militant workers' movement in the structures of state and polity as well as a growing acceptance of the social and economic functions of government rendered social regulation a less controversial issue, there still exist troubling traces of how thoroughly contagion has limited the possibilities of individual liberty. As late as the 1960s, the medical verification of sexually transmitted diseases remained a central component in the police regulation of prostitution in Paris.[6] As anxiety about the problem of poverty began to subside, the category of contagion informed new social dangers in need of government regulation, manifested most prominently in the role assumed by scientific investigation and institutions in the government of French colonial territories.[7] But it was French intellectuals who, in the wake of the Paris student uprisings of 1968, began to bring to public attention how the daily preoccupation with "the social" (including, but not limited to, the problem of disease) had completely extinguished the possibility of individual and collective political engagement that was so much a part of the late-eighteenth- and nineteenth-century Republican legacy of individual liberty.[8]

Ironically (and in what amounts to a telling example of the power and effectiveness of scientific discourse), neither the lingering traces of the relationship between social regulation and the transformation of liberty nor the attempts by intellectuals to address and understand that relationship have prevented policy makers or the public from grounding their ideas about social regulation in the language of individual rights. In the late-twentieth-century debate over the uncertain future of social welfare systems in Western industrial nations, participants argue for and against its continued existence as a matter of rights, whether it be to defend the rights of children, the rights of mothers, the rights of the poor, or the rights of individuals from government intervention. More often than not, these arguments are supported by scientific evidence of disease—the unwed, substance-abusing mother with AIDS and the homeless man who carries the drug-resistant tuberculosis bacillus are just two of the most common images that are invoked, in contradictory ways, to support divergent interpretations of the relationship between rights and social regulation. These debates take into account neither the historical origins of social regulation, which was premised upon extending the role of governmental intervention in social life by denying and surpassing the link between social questions (like poverty) and rights, nor how the role of science in explaining and addressing social questions was instrumental to this political process that sought an alternative to the conflict-ridden category of rights as a source of social order.

By way of conclusion, I want to suggest that discussions about social welfare should begin by reconsidering these origins. In doing so, my intention is neither to argue for the continued existence of so-cial reform as it presently exists (now, as in the nineteenth century, it links the development of government intervention to the definition of individuals in terms of dangerous social groups and social prac-tices), nor to call for its wholesale dismantling (it at least had the vir-tue of prescience by recognizing that the exercise of political rights alone would not lead to social harmony and happiness). Rather, situ-ating contemporary concerns about social reform in a historical con-text will help to avoid the positing of arguments in terms of the time-less natural rights of individuals and universal scientific truths that of-ten only serve to conceal political strategies, justify existing social ine-qualities and suffering, and leave unexamined the operations of gov-ernmental intervention. To recognize the origins of social regulation as a response to the problem of rights is not to deny the value of indi-vidual rights and liberty. Rather, it is to recognize that the concept and practice of liberty take shape in specific, and often highly politi-cized, social contexts. Nor will a focus on these origins reject the truth value of science. Instead, it will reveal how the methods and aims of scientific activity are shaped by social concerns and interests. Once these connections are acknowledged, science can work more self-consciously and effectively to produce the social conditions necessary for the realization of liberty.[9]

*Reference Matter*

# Notes

## List of Abbreviations

AN   National Archives, Paris
APP  Archives of the Prefecture of Police, Paris
AS   Archives of the Department of the Seine, Paris

## Introduction

1. See generally, Accampo, Fuchs, and Stewart, *Gender and the Politics of Social Reform in France*; Elwitt, *The Third Republic Defended*; Hatzfeld, *Du paupérisme à la sécurité sociale*; Mitchell, *The Divided Path*; Stone, *The Search for Social Peace*.

2. Procacci, *Gouverner la misère*; Procacci, "Sociology and Its Poor"; Ewald, *L'État providence*.

3. For an analysis of the problem of rights and its relationship to social conflict, see Procacci, *Gouverner la misère*; and Sewell, *Work and Revolution in France*. Useful general histories of the Revolution of 1848 include Agulhon, *La République au village*; Agulhon, *1848 ou l'apprentissage de la république*; Amann, *Revolution and Mass Democracy*; Gossez, *Les Ouvriers de Paris*; Merriman, *The Agony of the Republic*; Price, *The French Second Republic*; Tilly and Lees, "Le Peuple de juin 1848."

4. See Coffin, "Social Science Meets Sweated Labor"; Scott, "A Statistical Representation of Work," in *Gender and the Politics of History*, pp. 113–38; Schafer, *Children in Moral Danger*.

5. d'Eichthal, *La Solidarité sociale*, p. 6. I want to thank Joan Scott for this ref-

erence. For a history of solidarism, see Hayward, "The Official Social Philosophy of the French Third Republic"; and Nicolet, *L'Idée républicaine en France*.

6. There are many excellent studies of Pasteur and the development of microbiology. See esp. Dagognet, *Méthodes et doctrines dans l'oeuvre de Pasteur*; De Kruif, *Microbe Hunters*; Dubos, *Louis Pasteur*; Duclaux, *Pasteur*; Geison, *The Private Science of Louis Pasteur*; Latour, *Les Microbes*; Salomon-Bayet, *Pasteur et la révolution pastorienne*.

7. Quoted in *Annales d'hygiène publique et de médecine légale*, 3d. ser., 29 (1892): 206–8.

8. See esp. Pelling, *Cholera*, and Latour, *Les Microbes*.

9. In *The Foul and the Fragrant*, the historian Alain Corbin has suggested the importance of contagion to the "pre-Pasteurian" miasma theory of disease: "The air of a place was a frightening mixture of the smoke, sulfurs, and aqueous, volatile, oily and saline vapors that the earth gave off and occasionally, the explosive material that it emitted, the stinking exhalations that emerged from the swamps, minute insects and their eggs, spermatic animalcules and far worse, the contagious miasmas that rose from decomposition" (pp. 12–13). I will discuss the importance of Villermé's work for the early-nineteenth-century conception of contagion in Chapter 1.

10. For recent works that emphasize this relationship between scientific rationality and the Republican promise of individual liberty, see Nord, *The Republican Moment*, chap. 2; and Nicolet, *L'Idée républicaine en France*.

11. The classic statement of this understanding of contagion is Ackerknecht, "Anticontagionism Between 1821 and 1867." His thesis has been challenged in recent years. See esp. Pelling, *Cholera*; and Cooter, "Anticontagionism and History's Medical Record." Pelling's book was an attempt to provide compelling evidence for a scientific understanding of contagion before Pasteur. Cooter aimed at rejecting an epistemology premised upon boundaries between science and politics that, in his view, informed the work of both Ackerknecht and Pelling.

12. I have found Michel Foucault's work helpful in conceptualizing the relationship between the human sciences and the development of the modern practices and objectives of government. See esp. *The Birth of the Clinic*, and "Governmentality." On the theme of science and the state in Old Regime and Revolutionary France more generally, see Baker, *Condorcet*; Baker, "Science and Politics at the End of the Old Regime"; Gillispie, *Science and Polity in France*; Rosanvallon, *L'État en France*; Rosen, "Cameralism and the Concept of Medical Police." For parallel developments in England, see Shapin and Schaffer, *Leviathan and the Air-Pump*.

13. Bk. 1, chap. 1, sec. 6, p. 4. For the importance of John Locke to the French Enlightenment, see Voltaire's *Philosophical Letters*, Letter 13, "On Mr. Locke," pp. 52–59.

14. This is best demonstrated by Foucault, *Birth of the Clinic*.
15. Jean-Jacques Rousseau, *The Social Contract*.
16. The term is Foucault's. See *Birth of the Clinic*, p. 35. For a brief history of the Academy of Medicine, see Gillispie, *Science and Polity in France*, pt. 2, chap. 3, and Hanaway, "Medicine, Public Welfare and the State."
17. Cabanis, *Rapports du physique et du moral de l'homme*, esp. the fifth *mémoire*, "De l'influence des sexes sur le caractère des idées et des affections morales," p. 311.

A sensitivity which profoundly retains the impressions of objects and from which results lasting determinations suits the role of the man. But a more volatile sensitivity which permits impressions to follow one another in rapid succession and which always allows the last one to dominate is the only [kind of sensitivity] suited to the role of women. Change this order, and the moral world will no longer be the same. In effect, the system of attachments depends almost entirely on social relations, and all civil societies take as the necessary basis for their regulation the primordial society of the family.

On Cabanis more generally, see Baker, "Closing the French Revolution"; Fraisse, *Reason's Muse*; Goldstein, *Console and Classify*, chap. 2; Gusdorf, *Les Sciences humaines*, pt. 2, secs. 1–3; Murphy, "Medical Knowledge and Statistical Methods"; Staum, *Cabanis*; Williams, *The Physical and the Moral*.

18. For very suggestive analyses of the construction of reason as it informed the development of the human sciences, see, Hacking, *The Taming of Chance*; and Daston, "Rational Individuals v. Laws of Society," in Krüger et al., *The Probabilistic Revolution*, pp. 295–304.

19. Surveys of hygiene institutions both in Paris and nationally include Ramsey, "Public Health in France"; and La Berge, *Mission and Method*.

20. For the enduring presence of the working-class dwelling in discussions about disease and social regulation more generally, see Shapiro, *Housing the Poor of Paris*; and Foucault, *Politiques de l'habitat*.

21. Among the many works that I have found helpful, see Cole, "The Power of Large Numbers"; Engelstein, *The Keys to Happiness*; Haraway, *Primate Visions*; Pedersen, *Family, Dependence, and the Origins of the Welfare State*; Riley, *"Am I that Name?"*; Schafer, *Children in Moral Danger*; Scott, *Gender and the Politics of History*; Scott, *Only Paradoxes to Offer*; Shapiro, *Breaking the Codes*.

22. A good example of this traditional approach is La Berge, *Mission and Method*. For the classic example of the revolutionary influence of Pasteur on public health, see De Kruif, *Microbe Hunters*. Even those historians who admit the importance of politics still continue to emphasize the boundaries between science and politics. For them, the important question is to under-

stand how and why politics impeded the diffusion, acceptance, and implementation of scientific truth in social life. See Murard and Zylberman, *L'Hygiène dans la république*; and Shapiro, *Housing the Poor of Paris*. For Germany, a similar approach can be found in Evans, *Death in Hamburg*.

### Chapter 1

1. For a history of the cholera epidemic of 1832, see Bourdelais and Raulot, *Une Peur bleue*; Chevalier, *Le Choléra*; Delaporte, *Disease and Civilization*; Kudlick, *Cholera in Post-Revolutionary Paris*; Sussman, "From Yellow Fever to Cholera."

2. An excellent portrayal of the efforts of hygienists and hygiene institutions on the eve of the cholera epidemic can be found in Corbin, *The Foul and the Fragrant*.

3. Boulay de la Meurthe, *Histoire du choléra-morbus*; Corbin, *The Foul and the Fragrant*, p. 159.

4. On the role of hospitals during the cholera epidemic, see Sussman, "From Yellow Fever to Cholera," pp. 253, 270–77. Mortality and morbidity statistics are provided by Kudlick, *Cholera in Post-Revolutionary Paris*, pp. 1–2.

5. The history of social change and conflict between 1820 and 1840 is well presented in Sewell, *Work and Revolution in France*; and Aguet, *Les Grèves*. For a local case study with important implications for understanding these national developments, see Bezucha, *The Lyon Uprising of 1834*. On the Revolution of 1830, see David Pinkney, *The French Revolution of 1830*.

6. Sussman, "From Yellow Fever to Cholera," pp. 283–84.

7. Kudlick, *Cholera in Post-Revolutionary Paris*, pp. 183–92; Sussman, "From Yellow Fever to Cholera," pp. 278–309.

8. See Delaporte, *Disease and Civilization*, esp. chaps. 5–7; Foucault, *Birth of the Clinic*; Goldstein, *Console and Classify*, chaps. 2, 3.

9. The question of determinism and how it related to the definition of the individual is explored in Hacking, *The Taming of Chance*; and Daston, "Rational Individuals v. Laws of Society."

10. On Broussais, see Foucault, *Birth of the Clinic*; and Ackerknecht, "Broussais." I have written more extensively on the work of Bichat and Bernard as part of a larger "Science of Man" in my dissertation, "Contagious Disease and Urban Government," chap. 1. Crucial works by Bichat in regard to these questions include *Anatomie générale*, 2 vols.; *Anatomie pathologique*; *Recherches physiologiques sur la vie et la mort*. For Bernard, see *Introduction à l'étude de la médecine expérimentale* and *Principes de médecine expérimentale*. In addition to the books cited above, I have found the following secondary works extremely helpful in thinking about Bichat, Bernard, and the "Science of Man": Conry, "Le Point de vue de la médecine expérimentale"; Dobo and Role, *Bichat*; Canguilhem, *Études d'histoire et de philosophie des sciences, Le*

*Normal et le pathologique*, and "Puissance et limites de la rationalité en médecine"; Grmek, "La Conception de la maladie"; Holmes, *Claude Bernard and Animal Chemistry*; Lesch, *Science and Medicine in France* and "The Paris Academy of Medicine and Experimental Science"; Maulitz, *Morbid Appearances*; Olmsted and Olmsted, *Claude Bernard and the Experimental Method*; Poupa, "Le Problème de l'évolution chez Claude Bernard; Schiller, *Claude Bernard et les problèmes scientifiques*.

11. Quoted in Kudlick, *Cholera in Post-Revolutionary Paris*, p. 78.

12. Bourdelais and Raulot, *Une Peur bleue*, p. 72.

13. On government policy during the yellow fever scare, see Sussman, "From Yellow Fever to Cholera," chaps. 1–2.

14. The full title of the completed report was: *Rapport sur la marche et les effets du Choléra-Morbus dans Paris et les communes rurales du Département de la Seine*. A detailed analysis of the commission's efforts can be found in Delaporte, *Disease and Civilization*, esp. chap. 4; and Sussman, *From Yellow Fever to Cholera*, pp. 329–50.

15. Bernard wrote: "It is the individual who always concerns the doctor. He is not the doctor of the human species, he is the doctor of the individual who exists in particular circumstances." Bernard, *Principes de médecine expérimentale*, p. 142.

16. Corbin, *The Foul and the Fragrant*, p. 31.

17. That term can be found in *Rapport sur la marche*, p. 123.

18. For a fuller discussion of the problem of rights, see Procacci, *Gouverner la misère*, "Sociology and Its Poor"; and Sewell, *Work and Revolution in France*.

19. *Rapport sur la marche*, p. 121.

20. On the relationship of work to citizenship and social order, see Procacci, *Gouverner la misère*, pp. 45–55.

21. *Rapport sur la marche*, chap. 8.

22. Ibid., p. 126.

23. Ibid., p. 124.

24. Mary Poovey has noted a similar association between the poor and their living space in the work of the British doctor and social investigator James Phillips Kay (later Kay-Shuttleworth, 1804–77): "[K]ay obscures impoverished individuals by aggregating the poor and assimilating them to the houses and neighborhoods they inhabit. This aggregation tends to spatialize the poor, so that when good individuals explore urban neighborhoods, they also authorize forays into domestic interiors and investigations of bodily processes like eating and sleeping. Personifying houses, as Kay does here, further transfers agency from the aggregated poor to social investigators, even though it remains unclear whether the outstretched arms plead for help or extend a contaminating embrace." "Anatomical Realism

and Social Investigation in Early Nineteenth-Century Manchester," in *Making a Social Body*, p. 82.

25. *Rapport sur la marche*, pp. 194–95.

26. Ibid., p. 198. For a comprehensive analysis of the relationship between disease and housing reform, see Shapiro, *Housing the Poor of Paris*.

27. The term is taken from Delaporte, *Disease and Civilization*, p. 86.

28. A history of the role of the Academy and an analysis of the investigations of social problems that it commissioned in the 1830s and 1840s can be found in Rigaudias-Weiss, *Les Enquêtes ouvrières en France*. Many recent works have focused on Villermé and the *Tableau*. A necessary starting point is Coleman, *Death Is a Social Disease*. See also, Lynch, *Family, Class, and Ideology in Early Industrial France*; Reddy, *The Rise of Market Culture*, pp. 169–80; Sewell, *Work and Revolution in France*, pp. 223–32.

29. For a history of Lyon silkworkers, see Bezucha, *The Lyon Uprising of 1834*.

30. Villermé, *Tableau*, 1:352–84.

31. Ibid., 1:vij.

32. Ibid., 2:244.

33. Ibid., 1:70.

34. Ibid., 2:47.

35. Bono, "Science, Discourse, and Literature," pp. 59–89.

36. Villermé, *Tableau*, 2: 38–39, 47.

37. Joan Scott has analyzed how references to women workers structured the explanations of poverty developed in these studies. See "L'Ouvrière! Mot impie, sordide . . . Women Workers in the Discourse of French Political Economy, 1840–1860," in *Gender and the Politics of History*, pp. 139–63.

38. Villermé, *Tableau*, 2:258.

39. Ibid., 2:219.

40. Ibid., 2:254.

41. For Villermé's intellectual and institutional kinship to Cabanis, see Coleman, *Death Is a Social Disease*, esp. pp. 126–31.

42. Villermé, *Tableau*, 2:257.

43. Ibid., 1:83. I am using Sewell's translation, *Work and Revolution in France*, p. 225.

44. Lynch, *Family, Class, and Ideology in Early Industrial France*, p. 192.

45. On this critical re-evaluation of political economy, see Procacci, *Gouverner la misère*, pts. 2 and 3.

46. In chapter 8 ("The Wages of Labor") of his *Wealth of Nations*, Smith argued that the increase in wealth causes a rise in wages, which in turn "increases the bodily strength of the laborer." Heilbroner, *The Essential Adam Smith*, p. 205.

47. Buret, *De la misère*, 2:171–72.
48. Ibid., 1:353.
49. Ibid., 1:380, 363. Adam Smith also invoked the Italian physician Ramazzini, but to provide evidence for the frequency of disease in economic systems that did not take as their basis the free accumulation of wealth. See note 46 above.
50. Buret, *De la misère*, 1:42.
51. Ibid., 2:318, 261.
52. Ibid., 1:406.
53. Ibid., 2:360.
54. Ibid., 1:416.
55. Ibid., 1:312–13.
56. Ibid., 2:321.
57. Ibid., 2:258.

## Chapter 2

1. Frégier, *Des classes dangereuses*, 1:269.
2. Ibid., 2:34–35.
3. Ibid., 2:29–30.
4. Ibid., 1:162, 370. On the gendering of social regulation, see Chapter 1.
5. Ibid., 2:222.
6. Ibid., 1:370. For an overview of the development of penal science and new practices of incarceration in nineteenth-century France, see O'Brien, *The Promise of Punishment*.
7. See Rosen, "Cameralism and the Concept of Medical Police."
8. Frégier, *Histoire*, 1:vi–vii.
9. Ibid., 1:525.
10. Ibid., 1:x.
11. The 1841 Child Labor Law, which preceded the 1850 Insalubrious Dwellings Law, was largely ineffective. See Schafer, *Children in Moral Danger*, p. 44.
12. For an early appreciation of the need for such a law, see the discussion of the official cholera report in Chapter 1. How the investigation of working-class conditions undertaken by Adolphe Blanqui (under the auspices of the Academy of Moral and Political Sciences) influenced this law is addressed by Procacci, *Gouverner la misère*, chap. 9.
13. On the Social Catholic movement in early-nineteenth-century France, see Lynch, *Family, Class, and Ideology in Early Industrial France*, esp. chap. 2. On the complex motivations behind this law more generally, see Danielle Rancière, "La Loi du 13 juillet 1850 sur les logements insalubres: Les Philanthropes et le problème insoluble de l'habitat du pauvre," in Foucault, *Politiques de l'habitat*, pp. 187–207.

14. The legislative history of the law was happily brief: It was deposed in July 1849, debated in March 1850, and enacted in April.

15. *Moniteur universel*, March 6, 1850, p. 785.

16. Ibid.

17. Ibid. , p. 786.

18. Ibid. , p. 787.

19. For a more detailed understanding of these prefectoral councils and how they represented state goals at the expense of local ones, see Bourdelais and Raulot, *Une Peur bleue*, chap. 7; and Murard and Zylberman, *L'Hygiène dans la république*, esp. pt. 3. A number of departments had created health councils before the 1848 law generalized them. Among the precursors were Nantes (1817), Lyon (1822), Marseille (1825), Lille (1828), Strasbourg (1829), Troyes (1830), Rouen and Bordeaux (1831), and Toulouse (1832). See La Berge, *Mission and Method*, p. 127.

20. Those legislative initiatives included the protection of infants (1874) and morally abandoned children (1889). See Cole, "The Power of Large Numbers"; and Schafer, *Children in Moral Danger*.

21. For Roussel's remarks, see *Moniteur universel*, March 6, 1850, p. 786–88.

22. The powers created by this law were intensively analyzed in a number of legal treatises and theses dealing with the regulation of disease immediately preceding and following the passage of the Public Health Law of 1902. I found the following particularly helpful: Garet, *Le Régime spécial de la ville*; Jouarre, *Des pouvoirs de l'autorité municipale*; Tréhu, *Des pouvoirs de la municipalité parisienne*.

23. For a comparison between these two laws, see the works listed in the preceding note. A good overview of the function of the prefecture of police can be found in O'Brien, "Urban Growth and Public Order."

24. On the activities of the prefecture of the Seine during the first half of the nineteenth century, see Jordan, *Transforming Paris*, chap. 4; Pinkney, *Napoleon III and the Rebuilding of Paris*, chap. 2; Sutcliffe, *The Autumn of Central Paris*.

25. These attributions of policing are laid out in great detail in administrative treatises. See esp. Block, *Dictionnaire de l'administration française*; Bouffet and Périer, *Traité du département*; de Pontich, *Administration de la ville de Paris*; Des Cilleuls, *Histoire de l'administration parisienne*, vol. 2; Sourdillon, *L'Autonomie communale à Paris*.

26. For a history of this repression, see Margadant, *French Peasants in Revolt*; and Merriman, *The Agony of the Republic*.

27. Quoted in Pinkney, *Napoleon III and the Rebuilding of Paris*, p. 38.

28. A comprehensive history of Haussmann's life and career can be found in Jordan, *Transforming Paris*.

29. Quoted in ibid., p. 130.

30. On the relationship between the extension of prefectoral attributes and the 1850 Insalubrious Dwellings Law (and disease regulation more generally), see Jordan, *Transforming Paris*, p. 113; Jouarre, *Des pouvoirs de l'autorité municipale*, pp. 110, 112–13, 139; Tréhu, *Des pouvoirs de la municipalité parisienne*, p. 14.

31. Haussmann relates this story in his *Mémoires*, pp. 6–10. See also Jordan, *Transforming Paris*, p. 212.

32. See the last section of this chapter, "Redefining Policing Under the Third Republic."

33. These statistics are taken from Jourdan, *Législation sur les logements insalubres*, pp. 178–80. Cities with other active commissions included Lille, Le Havre, Roubaix, and Nancy. See Murard and Zylberman, *L'Hygiène dans la république*, pp. 133–38.

34. AN F⁸ 213. Commission des logements insalubres. "Rapport général sur les travaux de la commission, 1860–1" (1863).

35. AN F⁸ 213. Commission des logements insalubres. "Affaires." Extract from an article that appeared in the *Annales d'hygiène publique et de médecine légale*, April 1881: "L'Eau est-elle nécessaire dans les habitations pour en assurer la salubrité?," p. 370.

36. AN F⁸ 211. Commission des logements insalubres. "Rapport général sur les travaux de la commission, 1862, 1863, 1864, 1865," (1866), p. 8.

37. See Sharon Marcus, *Apartment Stories*. In her analysis of Zola's *Pot-Bouille*, Marcus interprets Adèle's hiding of her newborn infant in a shared doorway as a symptom of an incomplete "interiorization," where the domestic realm threatens public order and public concerns are constantly impinging on the private space.

38. Tréhu, *Des pouvoirs de la municipalité parisienne*, p. 73. It is interesting to note, as a symptom of the conflict over attributions stemming from the problematic definition of insalubriousness, that another legal scholar, Jouarre, interpreted these dangers as regulated by the 1850 law.

39. AN F⁸ 213. On the Conseil d'état ruling, see Jourdan, *Études d'hygiène publique*, p. 188.

40. Tréhu, *Des pouvoirs de la municipalité parisienne*, pp. 91–92. In a letter to the minister of commerce dated July 1, 1850, the Comité consultatif d'hygiène publique wrote, "That which the law [of 1850] has not accomplished, the committee thinks the administration [prefecture of police] can do, at least to a certain extent, without exceeding the [legal] limits that are imposed on it." AN F⁸ 171. On the superior effectiveness of police powers, see also "Redefining Policing Under the Third Republic," below, and chap. 5.

41. This is the central theme of Tréhu's study. For cases in which landlords challenged the authority of the commission, see most importantly the investigation of the cité Jeanne d'Arc (1880–81), located in the thirteenth ar-

rondissement. Responding to the attempt by the commission to cite cases of smallpox in order to justify the imposition of fines, and perhaps even demolition, its landlord, M. Thuilleux, "rejects the competence of the Commission des logements insalubres by establishing a distinction between the causes of insalubriousness that would result from the defective disposition of spaces intended for habitation and that which would derive from the defect of the property itself." The latter, he argued, was under the jurisdiction of the prefecture of police, and thus the commission could not invoke cases of smallpox as the justification for its intervention. AN F⁸ 213. For an example of a case in which the prefecture of police was accused of overstepping its jurisdiction by "confusing property and salubriousness and by tending to substitute its action for the essentially free exercise of property," see the Affaire Delamotte (1859), AN F⁸ 213.

42. An excellent example of this is the Affaire cité Jeanne d'Arc. In invoking recurrent smallpox cases to justify its intervention, the commission quoted from an investigation undertaken by Dr. Delpech, a member of the Conseil d'hygiène publique.

43. For a detailed account of these events, see Pinkney, *Napoleon III and the Rebuilding of Paris*, chap. 8; and Jordan, *Transforming Paris*, chap. 13.

44. Barrows, *Distorting Mirrors*.

45. See Guillermond, *Les Services d'hygiène*, pp. 12–13. On criticism of the prefecture of police after the Commune, see Des Cilleuls, *L'Administration parisienne*; and Sourdillon, *L'Autonomie communale*.

46. See, for example, the debate on January 15, 1884. AN F⁸ 171. Prefect Andrieux's defense of his office at this session is discussed below.

47. Sourdillon, *L'Autonomie communale*, pp. 29–30.

48. On Parent-Duchâtelet and the regulation of prostitution more generally, see Corbin, *Women for Hire*. For the influence of Parent-Duchâtelet beyond France, see Engelstein, *The Keys to Happiness*, esp. chaps. 4, 5.

49. See Corbin, *Women for Hire*, pp. 220–30. The campaign against police regulation has been vividly recounted by Berlière, *La Police des moeurs*.

50. AN F⁸ 171. Chamber of Deputies, Session of January 15, 1884. "Première délibération sur le projet de loi tendant au rattachement au budget de l'état des dépenses de la police dans la ville de Paris (extract)."

51. Prefecture of police. "Note en réponse au mémoire de M. le Préfet de la Seine sur les attributions de la Préfecture de Police," pp. 8–9.

52. Ibid., p. 6.

53. AN F⁸ 171. Chamber of Deputies, Session of January 21, 1884 (extract).

54. Lépine et al., "Notions générales de police," pp. 4, 10.

55. Quoted in Berlière, *La Police des moeurs*, p. 83 (italics in original).

Chapter 3

1. Glanders, consumption, anthrax, septicaemia, and typhoid fever were just some of the diseases considered here. For an understanding of the structure and activities of the Academy of Medicine, I have relied upon Weisz, *The Medical Mandarins*.

2. For a re-evaluation of the debate over contagion and spontaneous generation, see Latour, "Pasteur et Pouchet."

3. *Bulletin de l'Académie de médecine* 26 (1860–61): 1022.

4. Ibid. 32 (1866–67): 1173–75.

5. Ibid. 15 (1849–50): 988.

6. Ibid. 29 (1863–64): 1081.

7. Ibid. 29 (1863–64): 1153.

8. Ibid., 2d ser., 13 (1884): 1296–99; 26 (1860–61): 1053. On the suggestion to create a nosological distinction between "typhoïde" and "typhoïdette," see Paul Brouardel, "Modes de propagation de la fièvre typhoïde," *Annales d'hygiène publique et de médecine légale*, 3d ser., 18 (1887): 398 (paper given before the 1887 International Congress of Hygiene and Demography at Vienna).

9. For a perceptive analysis of the centrality of language to the Scientific Revolution, see Bono, *The Word of God and the Languages of Man*.

10. *Bulletin de l'Académie de médecine* 29 (1863–64): 1013; 33 (1868): 492.

11. Ibid. 34 (1869): 295.

12. Ibid. 29 (1863–64): 1081.

13. Ibid. 2d ser., 2 (1873): 1282; 33 (1868): 240–41.

14. Ibid. 29 (1863–64): 1070.

15. Ibid. 32 (1866–67): 1249.

16. Ibid. 33 (1868): 247–48.

17. For an analysis of a related scientific debate that breaks down the distinction between knowledge and contextual factors, see Latour, "Pasteur et Pouchet."

18. *Bulletin de l'Académie de médecine*, 2d ser., 6 (1877): 653.

19. Ibid. 32 (1866–67): 1243.

20. Ibid. 2d ser., 7 (1878): 434–52.

21. See esp. Dagognet, *Méthodes et doctrines dans l'oeuvre de Pasteur*; De Kruif, *Microbe Hunters*; Dubos, *Louis Pasteur*; Duclaux, *Pasteur*; Geison, *The Private Science of Louis Pasteur*; Latour, *Les Microbes*; Salomon-Bayet, *Pasteur et la révolution pastorienne*.

22. According to Dagognet, "Pasteur only deepens the chasm separating the 'mineral' and the 'vital,' death and life." *Méthodes et doctrines*, p. 69.

23. "All the chemistry treatises of the eighteenth and nineteenth centuries took as identical fermentation and illness. Since Pasteur studied the first, he found himself naturally directed toward the second." *Méthodes et doctrines*, pp. 167–68.

24. On these developments I have found useful the works by Dagognet, *Méthodes et doctrines*, pp. 4–67; and Geison, *The Private Science of Louis Pasteur*, chaps. 3, 4.

25. See note 23, above.

26. In this regard, the comment of Pasteur's student and biographer Émile Duclaux is especially illuminating: "La Levure est un être comme vous." *Pasteur*, p. 96.

27. Duclaux wrote extensively on how morbid exteriority improved upon physiological conceptions of a virus whose functions, defined by and thus inseparable from the body, were inaccessible to scientific investigation and explanation. See his *Traité de microbiologie* 1:30–31. See also Dagognet, *Méthodes et doctrines*, pp. 216, 225.

28. For one example of this, see Bouillaud's comment, p. 77. On anthrax and its importance for Pasteur's work, see Dagognet, *Méthodes et doctrines*, pp. 182–88; Duclaux, *Pasteur*, pp. 294–328; Geison, *The Private Science of Louis Pasteur*, chap. 6. What follows is based upon the analyses developed in these works.

29. Geison, *The Private Science of Louis Pasteur*, p. 145.

30. Duclaux, never one to underestimate the revolutionary nature of his mentor's achievements, is particularly effective on Pasteur's investigation of anthrax. *Pasteur*, pp. 304–19.

31. The two best accounts of the experiments at Pouilly-le-Fort are Latour, *Les Microbes*, pp. 95–103; and Geison, *The Private Science of Louis Pasteur*, chap. 6. Their analyses, however, are very different. As a sociologist of knowledge, Latour argues that the brilliant success of Pasteur's demonstration was dependent upon things usually considered "outside" the laboratory, in the end rendering it impossible to make distinctions between the space, methods and goals of the laboratory, and the social world. Geison's approach, discussed immediately below, admits that "outside factors"—most notably professional ambition—shaped Pasteur's demonstration at Pouilly-le-Fort. It does so, however, without rejecting the epistemology that defines scientific knowledge and the social world as distinct and separate.

32. Geison, *The Private Science of Louis Pasteur*, p. 14.

33. Duclaux's explanation of the variation of virulence suggests how this concept challenged the definition of the microbe as a specific cause: "If the *espèce* were immutable, there would be no other *êtres* worthy of carrying the specific name except for those which possess the same properties. Experimentation shows that this is not so and that, around this *être typique*, are placed and ordered a crowd of other *êtres*, some of which no longer have the properties which formed the basis of definition, while all the time preserving with the preliminary [*espèce*] the bond of a regular filiation." *Traité de microbiologie* 1:261.

34. *Bulletin de l'Académie de médecine*, 2d ser., 7 (1878): 440.

35. Ibid., 2d ser., 8 (1879): 1154.

36. For Bouillaud's comments, see ibid., pp. 1154, 1159.

37. See Fauvel's comments in discussions about typhoid fever, *Bulletin de l'Académie de médecine*, 2d ser., 12 (1883): 465.

38. On Koch's contributions and his rivalry with Pasteur, see Geison, "Pasteur," pp. 398–99. For a German historian's perspective on these developments, see Evans, *Death in Hamburg*.

39. Consider Gabriel Colin's comments on septicaemia: "It is not enough that germs, microscopic living things, soluble or figurative ferments that penetrate the organism, spread in the tissues or the fluids in order for accidents to be produced. The germs will only succeed in developing, the microscopic things in multiplying, if they find those conditions necessary for their evolution and existence." *Bulletin de l'Académie de médecine*, 2d ser., 8 (1879): 20–23.

40. This idea was best represented in the 1883 typhoid fever discussion at the Academy by Michel Peter. See below, pp. 84–87.

41. For a detailed description of this method, see Oriou, "Diagnostic précoce de la tuberculose: Calcul de la formule respiratoire chez l'homme par la méthode du Professor Créhant et par des mesures spirométriques," *Annales d'hygiène publique et de médecine légale*, 3d ser., 41 (1899): 424–524.

42. APP DB 458. See "Avis relatifs aux précautions à prendre contre le danger du charbon," "signed" by Bouchardat, Hillairet, and Pasteur (rapporteur) and read, adopted, and distributed by the Conseil d'hygiène publique et de salubrité, July 7, 1882.

43. *Cours d'hygiène professé à l'Institut d'hygiène à la faculté de médecine*, chap. 15, p. 213.

44. *Bulletin de l'Académie de médecine*, 2d ser., 8 (1879): 476–77.

45. Colin, *Traité des maladies épidémiques*, pp. 78–79.

46. Charrin, *Les Défenses naturelles de l'organisme*, p. 21.

47. Colin, *Traité des maladies épidémiques*, p. 94.

48. He published collectively his many reports for the Conseil and the Academy of Medicine in *Études d'hygiène publique*. These statistics were part of a report he undertook for the Academy of Medicine, "Les Épidémies de France, 1887–8," reproduced in 3:167.

49. This was Brouardel's comment to the pathologist Michel Peter during the 1892 debate over cholera. The positions of both individuals are discussed below in more detail. See *Bulletin de l'Académie de médecine*, 2d ser., 28 (1892): 575.

50. This concern was prominent in an investigation on the "transmission of consumption" undertaken by the Société médicale des hôpitaux, reprinted in *Revue d'hygiène* 8 (1886): 281.

51. These comments were delivered at a discussion of cholera that took place at the *Société de médecine publique*; summary of minutes reproduced in *Annales d'hygiène publique et de médecine légale*, 3d ser., 12 (1884): 355.

52. "La Contagion dans la rue," in *Annales d'hygiène publique et de médecine légale*, 3d ser., 12 (1884): 482.

53. See, for example, Administration générale de l'Assistance publique à Paris, "Commission spéciale instituée à l'effet d'étudier et de déterminer les mesures propres à empêcher la contagion de la tuberculose" (1897). The members included the hygienist Brouardel, the clinicians and tuberculosis experts Joseph Grancher and Louis Landouzy, Pasteur Institute official Émile Roux, and Brouardel's protégé Léon Thoinot.

54. The 1903 report of the municipal (Paris) commission in charge of reviewing health regulations subtly suggested the complex interests involved in the question of isolating people with tuberculosis: "The administration cannot confine in isolation hospitals, similar to leper-hospitals, all those suffering from tuberculosis; these measures are excessive and hardly characteristic of our age." A copy of this report can be found in the prefecture of police archives, DB 457.

55. Ollivier was especially vociferous in calling for strict isolation techniques in hospitals treating childhood diseases like diphtheria, chicken pox, and scarlet fever. Among the measures he envisioned to transform the hospital into a *"colonie sanitaire,"* he advocated communication between parents and their isolated children via telephone. See his report for the Conseil d'hygiène publique et de salubrité, "Rapport sur la scarlatine, à Paris en 1886 et sur la prophylaxie générale des maladies contagieuses chez les enfants" (1887), as well as other reports collected in his *Études d'hygiène publique*. The role of parents in spreading disease will be considered more fully in Chapter 5. For the problem of hospital attendants who spread disease when frequenting the café Château des Alouettes outside the Aubervilliers hospital, see Georges Dujardin-Beaumetz's report for the Conseil d'hygiène publique et de salubrité, "Rapport sur les cas de variole observés dans les dix-huitième et dix-neuvième arrondissements" (1887).

56. "Tuberculose pulmonaire et sanatoriums," p. 30 (extract from *Bulletin médical*, March 7, 1903). For more on Grancher's social vision, see Murard and Zylberman, *L'Hygiène dans la république*, esp. chap. 16.

57. Bouchard, *Thérapeutique des maladies infectieuses*, p. 35.

58. Bouchard, *Leçons sur les auto-intoxications*, p. 275. Here, Bouchard refers to the self-experimentation of Bochefontaine, who "swallowed pills containing cholera evacuations [déjections]."

59. Ibid., pp. 202–3.

60. Ibid., p. 9.

61. Bouchard, *Thérapeutique des maladies infectieuses*, p. 102.

62. Ibid., pp. 293–94. Some salutary influences he mentioned for curing consumption/tuberculosis (he uses both nosological categories) were: "moral satisfaction, absence of worries, good distractions, exercise, contact with good air at high altitudes," p. 350.

63. Bouchard, *Leçons sur les auto-intoxications*, p. 16.

64. Ibid., p. 268. Here, Bouchard refers explicitly to cholera, and very likely the cholera epidemic of 1884, which initiated a lively and contentious debate on importation. The issue of importation is addressed in more detail in Chapter 4 and the introduction to Chapter 5.

65. Bouchard, *Thérapeutique des maladies infectieuses*, pp. 16–17.

66. Peter's reputation was defined by his participation in two debates that are particularly well documented in the proceedings of the Academy of Medicine: typhoid fever (1883) and cholera (1892).

67. For recent appraisals of Peter's work, see Latour, *Les Microbes*, pp. 35–38; and Geison, *The Private Science of Louis Pasteur*, pp. 220–29.

68. *Bulletin de l'Académie de médecine*, 2d ser., 13 (1884): 1124–25.

69. For a good example of how Peter conceived morbid spontaneity as a supplement to microbiology, see Ibid., 12 (1883): 413. In an example of his polemical style, Peter claimed that Pasteur himself had recognized the importance of morbid spontaneity.

70. Ibid., 2d ser., 12 (1883): 233.

71. Ibid., 2d ser., 28 (1892): 476.

72. Bouley's accusation was a response to Peter's criticism of the eminent physiologist Claude Bernard. Peter responded to the accusation thus: "Son of an Alsatian, I bear a German name, but my heart is profoundly French; no one is more or better aware of the greatness of my country. . . . I also admire Claude Bernard; but when Claude Bernard appears to me to be mistaken, I do not hesitate to reveal it." *Bulletin de l'Académie de médecine*, 2d ser., 12 (1883): 373.

73. The most comprehensive account of the developments of hygiene in the age of Pasteur is Murard and Zylberman, *L'Hygiène dans la république*. See also Latour, *Les Microbes*, pp. 22–35, 51–60. Latour argues for a process of reciprocal definition between hygienists and Pasteurian microbiologists, where hygienists provided an agenda and Pasteurians supplied the scientific technique (the laboratory). As I hope the following pages demonstrate, hygienists did much more than offer their long-standing goal of "assainissement des villes." They furnished methods for investigating the role of social conditions in the production of disease and in so doing surpassed the limitations of Pasteur's "morbid exteriority." Finally, while his work mainly focuses on the development of hygiene in the 1830s and 1840s, Bernard Lécuyer's "Probability in Vital and Social Statistics: Quételet, Farr and the Bertillons" (in Krüger et al., *The Probabilistic Revolution*, vol. 1, pp. 317–35)

offers some useful information on hygiene at the end of the nineteenth century.

74. Bouchardat, *Traité d'hygiène*, p. 1. This was the third edition of his treatise.

75. Monin, *La Lutte pour la santé*, p. 143.

76. Rochard, "L'Avenir de l'hygiène," p. 3.

77. See Chap. 4, below.

78. Reprinted in *Annales d'hygiène publique et de médecine légale*, 3d ser., 9 (1883): 274.

79. Although much larger than many of the other towns and cities he visited, Le Havre is a good example of this approach. Comité consultatif d'hygiène, "Enquête sur les causes d'épidémies."

80. Brouardel's articles are replete with references to his association with members of the elite of Parisian medical science. He both collaborated with Chantemesse (who held the hygiene chair on the Paris medical faculty and served as director of its bacteriological laboratory) and sent him water samples for testing. He also refers to cases of typhoid fever he observed and treated with Bouchard and Landouzy. See "Enquête sur une épidémie de fièvre typhoïde qui a regné à Pierrefonds en août et septembre 1886," *Annales d'hygiène publique et de médecine légale*, 3d ser., 17 (1887): 106; "Modes de propagation de la fièvre typhoïde: Conférence au Congrès d'hygiène et de démographie de Vienne, 1887," *Annales d'hygiène publique et de médecine légale*, 3d ser., 18 (1887): 421–22.

81. Brouardel et Chantemesse, "Enquête sur les causes de l'épidémie de fièvre typhoïde qui a regné à Clermont-Ferrand," *Annales d'hygiène publique et de médecine légale*, 3d ser., 17 (1887): 393; see also Comité consultatif d'hygiène, "Enquête sur les causes d'épidémies de fièvre typhoïde au Havre."

82. Brouardel et Chantemesse, "Enquête sur les causes de l'épidémie de fièvre typhoïde qui a regné à Clermont-Ferrand," p. 401.

83. Brouardel, "L'Étiologie de la fièvre typhoïde au Havre," *Annales d'hygiène publique et de médecine légale*, 3d ser., 31 (1894): 427, 452–53. On Gibert, see Murard and Zylberman, *L'Hygiène dans la république*, pp. 185–89.

84. Brouardel, "Modes de propagation de la fièvre typhoïde," p. 399.

85. Ibid., p. 399.

86. Brouardel, "L'Étiologie de la fièvre typhoïde au Havre," p. 453. For the debate between Brouardel and Gibert, see *Bulletin de l'Académie de médecine*, 2d ser., 30 (1894): 401–11.

87. Brouardel, "Des moyens de préserver l'Europe contre les maladies exotiques (peste, fièvre jaune, choléra)" (January 24, 1885), reprinted from *Annales d'hygiène publique et de médecine légale*, 3d ser., 30 (1885): 229–52.

88. Ibid., p. 252.

89. On solidarism, see J. E. S. Hayward, "The Official Social Philosophy

of the French Third Republic." In his contribution to *La Solidarité sociale*, d'Eichthal invokes contagion as part of his attempt to rearticulate the conception of individualism. See Introduction, note 5.

90. Brouardel, "La Propreté et l'hygiène," pp. 19–20.

91. Ibid. Brouardel offers a vivid and horrifying scenario: The wife and mother who accepts factory work does not have time to clean the house. Her husband, disgusted and threatened by his wife's absence, spends more time at the cabaret, where he either contracts or is made receptive to—Brouardel's analysis is unclear—tuberculosis. He consequently gets sick and spreads the disease to other family members through coughing and sullied sheets and clothing. Husband, wife, and children end up in the hospital, and all die. The narrative conventions of this story follow closely the analysis of poverty provided by Jules Simon, a Third Republic apologist and political economist whom Brouardel explicitly acknowledged in this article. On Simon and the gendered understanding of social problems, see Scott, "L'Ouvrière! Mot impie, sordide . . . Women Workers in the Discourse of French Political Economy, 1840–1860" in *Gender and the Politics of History*, pp. 139–63.

92. For how this contradiction shaped the possibilities of individualism and state regulation (and the relationship of women to both), see Scott, *Only Paradoxes to Offer*.

93. For the role of provincial scientists at the Academy, see Weisz, *The Medical Mandarins*, chap. 2.

94. Arnould, "Une petite épidémie de fièvre typhoïde à étiologie complexe," excerpted from *Revue d'hygiène et de police sanitaire* 13 (1891): 14.

95. Arnould, "Considérations sur l'atmosphère de la ville de Lille," *Annales d'hygiène publique et de médecine légale*, 3d ser., 1 (1879): 418–20.

96. Conseil d'hygiène du département du Nord, "Épidémie d'accidents gastro-intestinaux" (1893), p. 25.

97. Arnould, "L'Eau de boisson," p. 6.

98. Arnould, "Études d'étiologie," p. 9.

99. Arnould, "De la fièvre typhoïde à l'état sporadique, son importance au point de vue de l'hygiène et de l'étiologie," *Revue d'hygiène* 8 (1886): 754.

100. The book was written by "a rationalist, medical doctor from the Paris medical faculty." Arnould reviewed the book in *Revue d'hygiène* 8 (1886): 60–62.

101. Arnould, "Une petite épidémie," pp. 3–4.

102. Arnould, "Études d'étiologie," pp. 55–60.

103. Ibid., p. 35.

104. Arnould, "Une petite épidémie," pp. 17–18.

105. Arnould, "L'Hygiène ancienne."

106. Ibid., p. 13.

107. Ibid., p. 10.

108. Ibid., p. 13.

109. Ibid.

110. Kelsch, *Traité des maladies épidémiques*, p. 24.

111. Ibid., p. 402.

112. Ibid. pp. 382–86.

113. Kelsch, "Considérations critiques sur la contagion et l'origine des maladies infectieuses," *Bulletin de l'Académie de médecine*, 2d ser., 36 (1896): 758.

114. *Les Microbes*. While Latour situates hygienists and microbiologists in a network of interests and forces that effectively breaks down commonly held distinctions between scientific knowledge and contextual factors, he in the end makes it clear that microbiologists are both defined and empowered by the scientific methods and instruments that the ambitious, agenda-oriented hygienists lack and need. Kelsch is just one example of the need to re-evaluate Latour's schema. Kelsch found in hygiene the scientific methods that, in his view, would redress the incapacity of microbiology to consider the social conditions of microbial transmission. Of course, even as Kelsch invoked the scientific superiority of hygiene, he was pursuing a complex of professional and social interests that in many important ways confirms Latour's analysis.

115. Kelsch, "Quelques réflexions sur la pathogénie des affections tuberculeuses, d'après observations cliniques et anatomo-pathologiques," reprint of a paper delivered at the Academy of Medicine, February 7, 1893, p. 4.

116. Kelsch, *Traité des maladies épidémiques*, i–ii.

117. This comment was part of Kelsch's response to a report delivered at the Academy of Medicine by Dujardin-Beaumetz on the problem of typhus in prisons located in the department of the Seine. *Bulletin de l'Académie de médecine*, 2d ser., 29 (1893): 405–6.

118. For an analysis of the system of prizes organized by the Academy, see Weisz, *The Medical Mandarins*, chap. 4.

119. Kelsch offered these statistics as part of his response to Grancher's report on tuberculosis in *Bulletin de l'Académie de médecine*, 2d ser., 39 (1898): 636. For an understanding of Kelsch's army career, see Osborne, "French Military Epidemiology."

120. "Quelques réflexions sur la pathogénie et la prophylaxie de la tuberculose," p. 5.

121. He made this statement during the debate over typhus. *Bulletin de l'Académie de médecine*, 2d ser., 29 (1893): 410.

122. Ibid., p. 414.

123. A literal translation would be "everything into the sewer." The following pages rely heavily on Jacquemet, "Urbanisme parisien," pp. 505–48; and Guerrand, "La Bataille du tout-à-l'égout," pp. 66–74. See also Reid, *Paris Sewers and Sewermen*.

124. These figures are taken from Jacquemet, "Urbanisme parisien," pp. 518–20.

125. Ibid., pp. 538–39.

126. The legal issues raised by tout-à-l'égout, especially as they relate to prefectoral power, are superbly analyzed in Tréhu, *Des pouvoirs de la municipalité parisienne*.

127. Jacquemet, "Urbanisme parisien," p. 544.

128. See Reid, *Paris Sewers and Sewermen*, p. 62; and Jacquemet, "Urbanisme parisien," p. 548. After a sophisticated political analysis of the multiple and conflicting interests that shaped this debate, Jacquemet suddenly poses the question of the scientific effectiveness of tout-à-l'égout: "On ne peut nier cependant qu'en poussant le tout-à-l'égout a provoqué une amélioration notable de la salubrité des habitations et a conduit les individus à prendre des habitudes d'hygiène corporelle dont les travaux de Pasteur ont montré qu'elles étaient essentielle pour le maintien d'une bonne santé. Ce n'est pas le moindre paradoxe que Pasteur, adversaire déterminé du tout-à-l'égout, ait, par sa propre activité scientifique, prouvé qu'il était nécessaire." The point of my argument here is that one cannot extract either the ideas or the actions of scientists from the political and professional interests that Jacquemet—his comments on Pasteur notwithstanding—has so ably analyzed.

129. Discussion at the Société de médecine publique, March 22, 1882, minutes reprinted in *Annales d'hygiène publique et de médecine légale*, 3d ser. 7 (1882): 427.

130. See his comments at the March 22, 1882, meeting of the Société, minutes reprinted in *Revue d'hygiène* 4 (1882): 428; and at the March 25, 1885, meeting, minutes reprinted in *Revue d'hygiène* 7 (1885): 331.

131. March 25, 1885, meeting of the Société, minutes reprinted in *Revue d'hygiène* 7 (1885): 337.

132. March 22, 1882, meeting of the Société, minutes reprinted in *Annales d'hygiène publique et de médecine légale* 4 (1882): 427.

133. Quoted in Latour, *Les Microbes*, p. 64.

134. Quoted in Vallin, "Les Projets d'assainissement de Paris," *Revue d'hygiène* 3 (1881): 827. In this article, Vallin, the editor of the *Revue*, summarized the discussions of the ministerial "*commission mixte*" that was set up in 1880 to address the "*odeurs de Paris*."

135. Du Mesnil, "L'Épidémie de diarrhée cholériforme devant le Conseil Municipal de Paris et devant le parlement," *Annales d'hygiène publique et de médecine légale*, 3d ser., 28 (1892): 524.

136. For Pasteur's participation in these debates, see AN $F^8$ 208, Commission de l'assainissement de Paris, meeting of December 18, 1880; AN C3385, Commission supérieur de l'assainissement de Paris (prefectoral), meeting of June 10, 1885. His remarks at both meetings exhibit a similar strategy. He claimed that the germ theory as it applied to anthrax was incontestable, although he admitted that sound scientific proof for extending it to other diseases

did not yet exist. However, since in his expert estimation the germ theory would be demonstrated for other diseases, he thought it only prudent to adopt a program for sewers that would prevent the possibility of transmission (namely, to reject tout-à-l'égout). To raise the stakes, Pasteur renounced any responsibility for the consequences that might ensue if that system were adopted.

137. AN F⁸ 208. Commission de l'assainissement de Paris. "Rapport sur les causes de l'infection signalée dans le département de la Seine pendant l'été 1880" (1881 draft, Brouardel, rapporteur), p. 63. For a fuller discussion of the term "foyer," see chaps. 4 and 5.

138. AN C5497. Préfecture du département de la Seine. "Direction des travaux de Paris." Commission technique de l'assainissement de Paris, minutes for meeting of December 23, 1882, p. 6.

139. The prefect of police removed Ulysse Trélat from the Conseil d'hygiène for refusing to take the oath to Napoleon III as stipulated by the constitution. He was replaced by Michel Lévy. See AN F⁸ 172.

140. See Shinn, *L'École polytechnique*, esp. chap. 4 and conclusion.

141. See Ellis, *The Physician-legislators*.

142. In ibid., p. 180, Ellis writes that "doctors evinced a deep tension between their hygienic idealism and the liberal ideology that characterized their social class. Few were eager to promote the cause of an intrusive state, and few liked the idea of higher taxes in order to implement public health laws."

*Chapter 4*

1. Colin, *Paris*, esp. pp. 183–85. For his analysis of the problem of the working-class dwelling in Paris, Colin draws upon the work of one of his colleagues, the hygienist Octave Du Mesnil. Du Mesnil, who was associated with the prefecture of the Seine and the Commission des logements insalubres, is best known for *L'Habitation du pauvre* (1890).

2. Ibid., pp. 335–36.

3. Ibid., p. 149.

4. Ibid., pp. 150–51.

5. This is best expressed by Colin's insistence that disease be considered "endemic" rather than "epidemic." He uses typhoid fever as an index of permanent social problems such as insalubrious housing, the growth of working-class population, and the increased presence of leisure activities in modern Paris. For a more thorough example of Colin's attempt to reconsider the terms "epidemic" and "endemic," see his *Épidémies et milieux épidémiques*.

6. See Lukes, *Émile Durkheim*, p. 9. I have found this work extremely helpful for understanding Durkheim's life. See also Anthony Giddens's excellent introduction to his edited collection *Durkheim on Politics and the State*, pp. 1–31.

7. Durkheim, *Suicide*, pp. 132, 146–47. *Suicide* was first published in 1897.

8. For one example, see note 5 above. Also see Chapter 3, pp. 79–80, 89.

9. The most comprehensive description of the operations of the Service des épidémies can be found in the official investigation (*enquête*) into the cholera epidemic of 1892, written and published by the Conseil d'hygiène publique et de salubrité in 1893. The purpose of this *enquête*, and others, was to explain and justify the administrative innovations in regulating disease. It is this relationship between explanation and administrative/political justification that will serve as the focus of this chapter. See Conseil d'hygiène publique et de salubrité, "L'Épidémie cholérique de 1892."

10. A full listing of his contributions would be impossible here. Most important, however, he edited and wrote the introduction to the general report of the Conseil (triennial by the 1880s), as well as the annual report summarizing the activities of the neighborhood hygiene commissions from 1889 until 1904, the very years of the Service's establishment and growth.

11. Léon Thoinot, *Histoire de l'épidémie cholérique de 1884*, p. 28.

12. See Conseil d'hygiène publique et de salubrité, "L'Épidémie cholérique de 1892," esp. pp. 37–38. The shelter appears to have included among its residents the infirm and poor as well as convicted criminals.

13. Préfecture de la Seine, Service de la Statistique Municipale (J. Bertillon, chef), "Tableaux statistiques de l'épidémie cholérique de 1884 à Paris et étude statistique des épidémies antérieurs" (1886), p. 14.

14. Conseil d'hygiène publique et de salubrité, "Rapport sur le typhus exanthématique à Paris," p. 44. A copy of this report can be found in the archives of the prefecture of police, DA 314.

15. Thoinot, *Histoire de l'épidémie cholérique de 1884*, p. 28.

16. Conseil d'hygiène publique et de salubrité, "Rapport général, 1890–94: Maladies contagieuses et épidémiques," p. 264.

17. Thoinot, *Histoire de l'épidémie cholérique de 1884*, p.62.

18. Netter, Thoinot, and Proust, "Le Choléra de la banlieue parisienne, de Paris et du département de la Seine et Oise en 1892 ...," *Bulletin de l'Académie de médecine*, 2d ser., 29 (1893): 270.

19. Brouardel, "Mortalité épidémique à Paris," *Annales d'hygiène publique et de médecine légale*, 3d ser., 8 (1882): 564.

20. It was Jeanne Gaillard who first discussed the relationship between the regulation of disease and the problem of the unsocialized poor and workers in modern Paris. See "Assistance et urbanisme dans le Paris du Second Empire," 395–422. On the anxiety produced by the homeless in nineteenth-century France, see also Perrot, "On the Fringe."

21. Thoinot, *Histoire de l'épidémie cholérique de 1884*, p. 29.

22. Ibid., p. 28. For an analysis of the role of Italian working-class immigrants in the 1884 epidemic and the fear they produced, see Snowden, *Naples in the Time of Cholera*, chap. 2, esp. pp. 65–66.

23. Conseil d'hygiène publique et de salubrité, "Rapport sur le typhus exanthématique à Paris," p. 53; Guérin coined the term "distribution vagabonde" to address the irregular patterns of transmission displayed during the 1884 cholera epidemic. See *Bulletin de l'Académie de médecine*, 2d ser., 14 (1885): 1019.

24. Conseil d'hygiène publique et de salubrité, "Rapport sur les asiles de nuit" (1893), p. 9.

25. On this law, see Sussman, "From Yellow Fever to Cholera," chap. 3.

26. Gaillard, "Assistance et urbanisme dans le Paris du Second Empire," p. 403.

27. The social problems posed by the transformation of Paris during the Second Empire are analyzed by Gaillard, *Paris, la ville*; and Clark, *The Painting of Modern Life*, chap. 1.

28. A good example of this can be found in Monod, *Le Choléra*, pp. 48–49. Monod's investigation of the origin of cholera in Concarneau led him to conclude it had been imported by local fishermen who had come into contact with a Spanish tuna boat. The local fishermen denied it, and Monod decided in the end to believe them, in part because he found regulatory measures that focused on local hygiene more effective and palatable than quarantines, which were usually adopted for "imported" or "exotic" diseases. Thoinot also gives the impression that oftentimes he had identified the elusive "immigrant" responsible for transmitting cholera in and around Toulon and Marseille in 1884. See *Histoire de l'épidémie cholérique de 1884*, p. 273.

29. Gaillard, "Assistance et urbanisme dans le Paris du Second Empire," p. 418.

30. Thoinot, *Histoire de l'épidémie cholérique de 1884*, p. 278.

31. The very best example of this was provided by Martellière, "De la fréquence et de la répartition de la fièvre typhoïde dans Paris." Martellière was the *rapporteur* for the neighborhood hygiene commission in the second arrondissement. In recognition of his acute observational skills, his 1882 report on typhoid fever, which under normal circumstances would have been summarized in the annual reports on the commissions' activity and on the incidence of epidemic disease reported to the prefecture, was published separately in 1884. A copy exists in the archives of the prefecture of police, DB 459.

32. Conseil d'hygiène publique et de salubrité, "Rapport sur les maladies épidémiques observées en 1883 dans le département de la Seine" (1885), pp. 12–14.

33. Martellière provided this example in "De la fréquence," pp. 34–35.

34. Ibid., p. 45.

35. *Bulletin de l'Académie de médecine*, 2d ser., 14 (1885): 1027–28; 13 (1884): 1579, 1669.

36. On the problem of rag-pickers in nineteenth-century France, see

Faure, "Classe malpropre, classe dangereuse?"; and Ratcliffe, "Perception and Realities of the Urban Margin."

37. *Bulletin de l'Académie de médecine*, 2d ser., 13 (1884): 1719.

38. "La Scarlatine sévit à Paris," *Le Matin*, July 27, 1907. A copy of this article can be found in the archives of the prefecture of police, DB 458.

39. Conseil d'hygiène publique et de salubrité, "Rapport sur les travaux des commissions d'hygiène du département de la Seine en 1883" (1885), p. 77.

40. Ibid., "Rapport sur les maladies épidémiques observées en 1879 dans le département de la Seine" (1881), p. 45.

41. Thoinot, *Histoire de l'épidémie cholérique de 1884*, p. 30.

42. Conseil d'hygiène publique et de salubrité, "Rapport général, 1887–9" (1889), p. 149.

43. Monod, *La Santé publique*, p. 7.

44. Conseil d'hygiène publique et de salubrité, "Rapport sur les travaux des commissions d'hygiène du département de la Seine en 1881" (1883), p. 93.

45. *Bulletin de l'Académie de médecine*, 2d ser., 22 (1889): 725.

46. Thoinot, *Histoire de l'épidémie cholérique de 1884*, p. 246.

47. Conseil d'hygiène publique et de salubrité, "Rapport sur les travaux des commissions du département de la Seine en 1890" (1892), p. 217.

48. The term "cry of alarm" was used by Gustave Jourdan, "Étude sur le projet de révision de la loi concernant les logements insalubres présenté à la Chambre des députés en 1883," in *Études d'hygiène publique*, p. 156.

49. The use of morbidity statistics to express national anxieties and rivalries can be found in the legislative record, cited below. See also the Senate report for a public health law, written in 1895 and presented in 1896. A copy is located in the archives of the prefecture of police, DB 454. For statistics as they relate to national comparisons, see Murard and Zylberman, *L'Hygiène dans la république*, chap. 12. On smallpox, see Darmon, *La Longue traque de la variole*. On the medicalized understanding of national decline during the Third Republic, see Nye, *Crime, Madness, and Politics in Modern France*.

50. Such pronouncements took many forms. They often materialized as hygienists and other members of the Academy of Medicine confronted difficult regulatory obstacles, the most serious being the cholera epidemic of 1884. Professional organizations such as the Société de médecine publique pursued the issue, and short articles and editorials on the topic of legislation were published in its journal *Revue d'hygiène*. The campaign for a public health law became identified, above all, with A. J. Martin, who served as inspector general for the Service de l'assainissement et de la salubrité de Paris. These organizations, and Martin in particular, played a formative role (largely mediated by the ministerial Comité consultatif d'hygiène publique) in the writing of the government project of law.

51. The legal scholar Léon Jouarre quoted Monod to underscore the impor-

tance that hygienists and interested parties in government regulation placed upon the efficacy and value of law: "Presently, salubriousness is at the discretion of individual and collective goodwill. In order for government authority to take charge of its defense, a law is necessary." *Des pouvoirs de l'autorité municipale*, p. 222.

52. Monod, *La Santé publique*, p. 6.

53. Two excellent histories of the process that produced the Public Health Law are Jourdan, *Législation des logements insalubres*; and Strauss and Fillassier, *Loi sur la protection de la santé publique*. Useful secondary sources include Carvais, "La Maladie, la loi et les moeurs," in Salomon-Bayet, *Pasteur et la révolution pastorienne*; Murard and Zylberman, *L'Hygiène dans la république*, chap. 4; Shapiro, *Housing the Poor of Paris*, chap. 6.

54. See esp. Murard and Zylberman, *L'Hygiène dans la république*; Shapiro, *Housing the Poor of Paris*.

55. *Journal officiel: Débats parlementaires, Sénat*, February 9, 1897, p. 133.

56. Ibid., February 12, 1897, p. 135.

57. This was Senator Buffet's response. Ibid., February 5, 1897, p. 97.

58. Ibid., February 4, 1897, p. 89.

59. Ibid., February 9, 1897, p. 132.

60. Ibid., February 4, 1897, p. 90.

61. *Journal officiel: Débats parlementaires, Chambre des députés*, June 26, 1893, p. 1836.

62. The colleague was Jolilos. Ibid., June 26, 1893, p. 1840.

63. Ibid., June 26, 1893, p. 1841; *Sénat*, February 9, 1897, p. 130.

64. *Journal officiel: Débats parlementaires, Sénat*, February 12, 1897, p. 156.

65. Ibid.

66. Strauss, *La Croisade sanitaire*, p. 15. For an informative analysis of Strauss's role in Third Republic social reform, see Rachel G. Fuchs, "The Right to Life: Paul Strauss and the Politics of Motherhood," in Accampo et al., *Gender and the Politics of Social Reform*, pp. 82–105.

67. *Journal officiel: Débats parlementaires, Sénat*, February 12, 1897, p. 157: "Who are the preferred victims when an epidemic rages? They are the poor, the completely destitute [misérables]."

68. Ibid., February 9, 1897, p. 124.

69. For an understanding of the law, I have relied upon Jourdan, *Législation des logements insalubres*; and Strauss and Fillassier, *Loi sur la protection de la santé publique*.

70. See the analysis of article 12 of the law in Strauss and Fillassier, *Loi sur la protection de la santé publique*, p. 341.

71. The obligatory declaration of cases of contagious disease was only one part of a much larger law. Hygienists regarded it as flawed, both because it excluded tuberculosis and because it provided doctors with numerous opportunities to evade reporting their patients to the authorities. See Robert

Carvais, "Le Microbe et la responsabilité médicale," in Salomon-Bayet, *Pasteur et la révolution pastorienne*, pp. 219–75; Murard and Zylberman, *L'Hygiène dans la république*, chap. 10.

72. Not surprisingly, legal scholars tended to be more critical of the law than government officials like Jourdan, Strauss, and Fillassier. For a critical evaluation of the law, see Garet, *Le Régime spécial*. Looking back on the "bizarre" split of attributions between the two prefects that was confirmed by the passage of the 1902 law, Garet wrote: "This is why we should not be surprised that, next to the great works of sanitation [assainissement] and embellishment that transformed certain parts of the capital during the last century, other parts remained veritable foyers of infection," p. 117.

73. Quoted in ibid., p. 47.

74. Quoted in ibid., p. 65.

*Chapter 5*

1. Robert Carvais, "La Loi et les moeurs," in Salomon-Bayet, *Pasteur et la révolution pastorienne*, pp. 281, 284.

2. Murard and Zylberman, *L'Hygiène dans la république*; Shapiro, *Housing the Poor of Paris*, p. 154.

3. The term is Carvais's. "La Loi et les moeurs," p. 284.

4. For recent important attempts to rethink the function of law during the Third Republic, see Ewald, *L'État providence*, esp. book IV, chap. 2, "Droit social"; Schafer, *Children in Moral Danger*; Jones, *The French State in Question*; and Donzelot, *L'Invention du social*.

5. *Annales d'hygiène publique et de médecine légale*, 3d ser., 12 (1884): 163–65.

6. Ibid., p. 187.

7. *Bulletin de l'Académie de médecine*, 2d ser., 13 (1884): 1233.

8. *Annales d'hygiène publique et de médecine légale*, 3d ser., 12 (1884): 189–90. For this excellent and well publicized example of Strauss's optimism, see his *La Croisade sanitaire*, p. 1.

9. For the analysis of this decree, I used the 1878 reprint of the instructions for implementation that the prefect of police sent to the commissions on September 23, 1852, APP DA 36.

10. AS V^bis 15 15^1, May 28, 1862.

11. AS V^bis 15 15^1, May 29, 1873.

12. AS V^bis 5.I^5 1, November 21, 1853.

13. AS VD^6 370, February 11, 1861. On this move from assistance to a politics of integration to be undertaken by the neighborhood commissions, see Gaillard, "Assistance et urbanisme dans le Paris du Second Empire."

14. AS VD^6 779, June 5, 1878.

15. AS VD^6 370, March 14, 1859.

16. The logic behind the choice of these four commissions was "diversi-

ty." The first and the fourth arrondissements were old and crowded, conjuring up the image of insalubriousness that spurred on the transformation of Paris. The fifth arrondissement was very poor and remained at the periphery of Haussmannization. The fifteenth arrondissement was a former "inner" suburb, incorporated only in 1860 and sparsely populated.

17. For a good overview of the diversity of Paris during the Second Empire and beyond, see Sutcliffe, *The Autumn of Central Paris*.

18. AS VD$^6$ 370, April 14, 1859 (correspondence).

19. AS VD$^6$ 370, February 16, 1853 (correspondence). Many of the neighborhood commissions were divided into sections responsible for investigating and reporting upon specific quarters.

20. AS V$^{bis}$ 5.I$^5$ 2, April 30, 1872.

21. AS VD$^6$ 779, June 5, 1878.

22. AS V$^{bis}$ 15 I$^5$ 1, February 28, 1861.

23. AS VD$^6$ 370, December 11, 1860.

24. AS V$^{bis}$ 4I$^5$ 4, March 21, 1872.

25. AS V$^{bis}$ 4I$^5$ 3, November 19, 1868.

26. AS V$^{bis}$ 5.I$^5$ 2, December 17, 1872.

27. AS VD$^6$ 779, September 8, 1877; and November 17, 1877.

28. AS VD$^6$ 370, June 12, 1860 (his emphasis).

29. AS V$^{bis}$ 5$^I$ 5$^2$, June 3, 1878.

30. Reprinted in his *Études d'hygiène publique*, vol. 2, pp. 11–139.

31. AS VD$^6$ 1344, November 8, 1882.

32. Ibid.

33. Conseil d'hygiène publique et de salubrité, "Rapport sur les travaux des commissions d'hygiène du département de la Seine en 1884" (1886), p. 26.

34. Conseil d'hygiène publique et de salubrité, "Comptes rendus" (1897), p. 477.

35. *Bulletin de l'Académie de médecine*, 2d ser., 11 (1882), p. 1259.

36. AS V$^{bis}$ 1I$^5$ 1, November 20, 1895.

37. See, for example, Kudlick, *Cholera in Post-Revolutionary Paris*, p. 113.

38. APP DB 458, Conseil d'hygiène publique et de salubrité, "Instructions: Choléra."

39. Conseil d'hygiène publique et de salubrité, "Rapport sur les travaux des commissions d'hygiène du département de la Seine en 1888" (1890), p. 213.

40. Conseil d'hygiène publique et de salubrité, "Rapport sur les travaux des commissions d'hygiène du département de la Seine en 1891" (1893), p. 132.

41. Conseil d'hygiène publique et de salubrité, "Rapport sur les travaux des commissions d'hygiène du département de la Seine en 1887" (1888), p. 149.

42. AS VD$^6$ 780 1, July 1, 1883.

43. AS VD$^6$ 1234, July 19, 1883.

44. On Bertillon, see Cole, "The Power of Large Numbers"; and Ber-

nard-Pierre Lécuyer, "Probability in Vital and Social Statistics: Quételet, Farr, and the Bertillons," in Krüger et al., *The Probabilistic Revolution*, pp. 317–35.

45. Conseil d'hygiène publique et de salubrité, "Rapports, 1892–4" (1895), pp. 25–31.

46. Conseil d'hygiène publique et de salubrité, "Rapport sur les maladies épidémiques observées dans le département de la Seine en 1879" (1881), p. 16.

47. AS VD⁶ 780 1, April 11, 1883.

48. AS VD⁶ 1344, December 19, 1882.

49. AS Vᵇⁱˢ 1I⁵ 1, November 17, 1897.

50. This term is taken from Elwitt, *The Making of the Third Republic*.

51. APP DB 458, Conseil d'hygiène publique et de salubrité, "Instruction populaire: Choléra" (1853). For a more detailed discussion of instructions for cholera, see Kudlick, *Cholera in Post-Revolutionary Paris*, pp. 105–16.

52. Moulin, *Hygiène et traitement du choléra-morbus: Coup d'oeil historique sur l'épidémie de Paris de 1832* (1832), p. 15. A copy can be found in APP DB 458.

53. APP DA 306 (1865).

54. For more details on the miasmatic theory of disease, see Chapter 1.

55. I have borrowed this term from Louis Chevalier's classic work *Laboring Classes and Dangerous Classes in Paris*. Chevalier used many of the documents relating to cholera as the basis for his "sociological" understanding of the biological causes of poverty and working-class militancy. In doing so, he failed to take into consideration the discursive production of these texts, something I am attempting to do here.

56. APP DA 305, "Reports on People Stricken with Cholera" (1865).

57. AS VD⁶ 1347, "Choléra: Secours, 1865–6."

58. Ibid.

59. Conseil d'hygiène publique et de salubrité, "Rapport général, 1884–6," p. 542.

60. On the unreliability of symptoms in an early period of scientific transformation, see Foucault, *The Birth of the Clinic*, chap. 6.

61. Conseil d'hygiène publique et de salubrité, "L'Épidémie cholérique de 1892," pp. 115–16.

62. APP DA 312, "Presumed case of cholera, 1890."

63. Ibid.

64. Ibid.

65. APP DA 312, "Presumed case of cholera, 1891."

66. APP DA 311, "Presumed case of cholera, 1885."

67. Ibid.

68. APP DA 308, "Presumed case of cholera, August 21, 1883."

69. Conseil d'hygiène publique et de salubrité, "Rapport de la Commission de choléra," in "Rapport sur les maladies épidémiques" (1883), p. 1.

70. APP DB 458, Conseil d'hygiène publique et de salubrité, "Instruction sur les précautions à prendre contre la diphtérie" (1884).

71. AS V<sup>bis</sup> 15 I<sup>5</sup> 4, January 30, 1902.

72. Conseil d'hygiène publique et de salubrité, "Rapport sur les travaux des commissions d'hygiène du département de la Seine en 1881" (1883), p. 26.

73. Conseil d'hygiène publique et de salubrité, "Comptes rendus," p. 461.

74. AS VD<sup>6</sup> 1344, July 9, 1890.

75. Conseil d'hygiène publique et de salubrité, "Rapport sur les travaux des commissions d'hygiène du département de la Seine en 1888" (1890), p. 43; 1889 (1891), p. 153.

76. Conseil d'hygiène publique et de salubrité, "Comptes rendus" (1897), p. 462.

77. AS V<sup>bis</sup> 15 15<sup>2</sup>, July 24, 1890, June 25, 1891.

78. Conseil d'hygiène et de salubrité, "Rapport sur les travaux des commissions d'hygiène du département de la Seine en 1889" (1891), pp. 42–43.

79. AS V<sup>bis</sup> 15 I<sup>5</sup> 3, February 27, 1896.

80. AS VD<sup>6</sup> 1345, April 22, 1903.

*Conclusion*

1. Murard and Zylberman, *L'Hygiène dans la république*, p. 576.

2. Ibid., pp. 577–78.

3. On the interwar economy, see Sauvy, *Histoire économique de la France entre les deux guerres*. The changing relationship between an organized workers' movement and the French state has been analyzed by Robert Wohl. Of course, political, social, economic, and cultural integration began long before the war. For two very different, and equally fascinating, accounts of this process, see Tilly, "Did the Cake of Custom Break?" and *The Contentious French*; Weber, *Peasants into Frenchmen*.

4. See esp. Hatzfeld, *Du paupérisme à la sécurité sociale*.

5. On Condorcet's vision of the relationship between science and liberal government, see Baker, *Condorcet*.

6. Berlière, *La Police des mœurs sous la IIIème République*, p. 168: "Un âge d'or [de la surveillance de la prostitution] auquel il fut apparemment mis fin en 1960, quand la France ratifia la convention adoptée par l'ONU en décembre 1949 sur la répression et l'abolition de la traite des êtres humains et de l'exploitation de la prostitution d'autrui."

7. Moulin, "Patriarchal Science," and "The Pasteur Institutes Between the Two World Wars."

8. The necessary starting point here is Donzelot, *L'Invention du social*.

9. See Epstein, *Impure Science*. Epstein demonstrates the crucial role of grassroots AIDS activism in the shaping of AIDS research and therapies.

# Bibliography

Primary Sources

Administration générale de l'Assistance publique à Paris. "Commission spéciale instituée à l'effet d'étudier et de déterminer les mesures propres à empêcher la contagion de la tuberculose." Paris, 1897.

Arnould, Jules. "Études d'étiologie: Étiologie de la fièvre typhoïde." Excerpted from *Gazette médicale*, 4th ser., 4 (1875).

———. "L'Eau de boisson considérée comme véhicule des miasmes et des virus et comme auxiliaire de leur absorption par les voies digestifs: Étude critique d'hygiène." Excerpted from *Gazette médicale*, 4th ser., 3 (1874).

———. "L'Hygiène ancienne et l'hygiène moderne." Leçon d'ouverture du cours d'hygiène à la Faculté de médecine de Lille. Paris: Cusset, 1878.

———. *Nouveaux éléments d'hygiène*. 3d ed. Paris: J.-B. Ballière, 1895.

Bernard, Claude. *Introduction à l'étude de la médecine expérimentale*. Paris: Flammarion, 1984.

———. *Principes de médecine expérimentale*. Paris: Presses universitaires, 1987.

Bernard, Léon, and Robert Debré, eds. *Cours d'hygiène professé à l'Institut d'hygiène à la Faculté de médecine*. Paris: Masson, 1927.

Bichat, Xavier. *Anatomie générale appliqueé à la physiologie et à la médecine*. 2 vols. Paris: G. Steinheil, 1900–1901.

———. *Anatomie pathologique: Dernier cours de Xavier Bichat, d'après un manuscrit autographe de P-A Béclard*. Paris: J.-B. Ballière, 1825.

———. *Recherches physiologiques sur la vie et la mort*, 4th ed. Paris: Béchet jeune, 1822.

Block, Maurice. *Dictionnaire de l'administration française*, 4th ed. Nancy and Paris: Berger-Levrault, 1898.

Bouchard, Charles. "Essai d'une théorie de l'infection: Maladie, guérison, immunité, virus, vaccins." Paper given at Internationaler medicinischer Congress, Berlin, 1890. Berlin: A. Hirschwald, 1890.

———. "Étiologie de la fièvre typhoïde." Paper given at the Congrès médical international de Genève, 1877. Paris: F. Savy, 1877.

———. "Exposé des travaux scientifiques du Dr. Charles Bouchard." Paris: Pillet et Dumoulin, 1886.

———. *Leçons sur les auto-intoxications dans les maladies: Professées à la Faculté de médecine de Paris pendant l'année 1885.* Paris: F. Savy, 1887.

———. *Thérapeutique des maladies infectieuses, antisepsie . . . Cours de pathologie générale: Professé à la Faculté de médecine de Paris pendant l'année 1887–1888.* Paris: F. Savy, 1889.

Bouchardat, Apollinaire. *Traité d'hygiène publique et privée basée sur l'étiologie.* 3d ed. Paris: F. Alcan, 1887.

Bouffet, Gabriel, and Léon Périer. *Traité du département: Historique du département, préfet, auxiliaire du préfet, conseil de préfecture.* Paris: P. Dupont, 1893–95.

Boulay de la Meurthe, Henri. *Histoire du choléra-morbus dans le quartier de Luxembourg.* Paris: P. Renouard, 1832.

Brouardel, Paul. "La Propreté et l'hygiène." In *Les Applications sociales de la solidarité: Leçons professées à l'École des hautes études sociales*, edited by Budin et al. Paris: F. Alcan, 1904.

Brouardel, Paul, and Léon Thoinot. *La Fièvre typhoïde.* Paris: J.-B. Baillière, 1895.

Buret, Eugène. *De la misère des classes laborieuses en Angleterre et en France avec l'indication des moyens propres à en franchir les sociétés.* 2 vols. Paris: Paulin, 1840.

Cabanis, Pierre-Jean-Georges. *Rapports du physique et du moral de l'homme.* 2 vols. Paris: Bibliothèque choisie, 1830.

Charrin, A. *Les Défenses naturelles de l'organisme: Leçons professées . . . au Collège de France.* Paris: Masson, 1898.

Colin, Léon. "Discussion sur l'épidémie de choléra. 1: Le Choléra à Aubervilliers. 2: Influence de l'eau de boisson." Reprint of a paper given at the Academy of Medicine, Paris, December 2, 1884.

———. *Épidémies et milieux épidémiques.* Paris: J.-B. Ballière, 1875.

———. *Paris: Sa topographie—son hygiène—ses maladies.* Paris: G. Masson, 1885.

———. *Traité des maladies épidémiques: Origine, évolution, prophylaxie.* Paris: J.-B. Ballière, 1879.

Comité consultatif d'hygiène (Paul Brouardel and Léon Thoinot, rapporteurs). "Enquête sur les causes d'épidémies de fièvre typhoïde au

Havre et dans l'arrondissement du Havre en 1887–8." In *Recueil de travaux du Comité consultatif*, vol. 19. Melun: Imp. administrative, 1889.

Conseil d'hygiène du département du Nord (J. Arnould, rapporteur). "Épidémie d'accidents gastro-intestinaux observée à l'école normale d'instituteurs, à Douai." Lille: L. Danel, 1893.

Conseil d'hygiène publique et de salubrité du département de la Seine (Georges Dujardin-Beaumetz, rapporteur). "L'Épidémie cholérique de 1892 dans le département de la Seine." Paris: Chaix, 1893.

———. "Rapport général: Comptes rendus," 1897–.Paris.

———. "Rapport général sur les travaux du Conseil d'hygiène publique et de salubrité." Paris: Chaix, 1872–96.

———. (Auguste Ollivier, rapporteur). "Rapport sur la scarlatine à Paris en 1886 et sur la prophylaxie générale des maladies contagieuses chez les enfants." Paris: Chaix, 1887.

———. (Georges Dujardin-Beaumetz, rapporteur). "Rapport sur le typhus exanthématique à Paris et dans le département de la Seine en 1893." Paris: Chaix, 1893.

———. (Georges Dujardin-Beaumetz, rapporteur). "Rapport sur les asiles de nuit." Paris: Chaix, 1893.

———. (Georges Dujardin-Beaumetz, rapporteur). "Rapport sur les cas de variole observés dans les dix-huitième et dix-neuvième arrondissements." Paris: Chaix, 1893.

———. "Rapport sur les maladies épidémiques observées dans le département de la Seine." Paris: Chaix, 1881–90.

———. "Rapport sur les travaux des commissions d'hygiène du département de la Seine et des communes de St.-Cloud, Sèvres, et Meudon." Paris: Boucquin, 1877–92.

d'Eichthal, Eugène, ed. *La Solidarité sociale: Ses nouvelles formules*. Paris, Alphonse Picard et fils, 1903.

de Pontich, Henri. *Administration de la ville de Paris et du département de la Seine*. Paris: Guillaumin, 1884.

Des Cilleuls, Alfred. *L'Administration parisienne sous la troisième république*. Paris: Picard, 1910.

———. *Histoire de l'administration parisienne au xixème siècle*, vol. 2: *Période 1830–1870*. Paris: H. Champion, 1900.

Dubousquet-Laborderie, Dr. "Étude sur l'épidémie cholérique de la commune de St. Ouen-sur-Seine du 30 avril au 25 octobre 1892." Published paper presented before the Société de médecine et de chirurgie pratiques de Paris, November 17, 1892. Paris, 1893.

Duclaux, Émile. *Pasteur: Histoire d'un esprit*. Sceaux, France: Charaire, 1896.

———. *Traité de microbiologie*. 2 vols. Paris: Masson, 1898.

Dujardin-Beaumetz, Georges. "Sur l'épidémie cholérique qui a atteint la ville de Paris pendant le mois de novembre 1884." Reprint of a paper given at the Academy of Medicine, Paris, December 9, 1884.

Du Mesnil, Octave. *L'hygiène à Paris: L'habitation du pauvre*. Paris: J.-B. Ballière, 1890.

Durand-Claye, Alfred. *L'Épidémie de fièvre typhoïde à Paris en 1882, étude statistique*. Nancy: Berger-Levrault, 1883.

Durkheim, Émile. *Suicide: A Study in Sociology*. Translated by John A. Spaulding and George Simpson. New York: Free Press, 1951.

Fillassier, Alfred. *De la détermination des pouvoirs publics en matière d'hygiène*. 2d ed. Paris: J. Rousset, 1902.

Frégier, Honoré Antoine. *Des classes dangereuses dans la population des grandes villes et des moyens de les rendre meilleures*. 2 vols. Paris: J.-B. Ballière, 1840.

———. *Histoire de l'administration de la police de Paris depuis Philippe-Auguste jusqu'aux États Généraux de 1789*. 2 vols. Paris: Guillaumin, 1850.

Garet, Maurice. *Le Régime spécial de la ville de Paris en matière d'hygiène*. Paris: Bonvalot-Jouve, 1906.

Guillermond, Georges. *Les Services d'hygiène de la Ville de Paris en 1908*. Paris: Librairie médicale et scientifique, 1908.

Haussmann, Georges-Eugène. *Mémoires du Baron Haussmann*, vol. 2: *Préfecture de la Seine*. 3d ed. Paris: Havard, 1890.

Jouarre, Léon. *Des pouvoirs de l'autorité municipale en matière d'hygiène et de salubrité*. Paris: V. Girard et E. Brière, 1899.

Jourdan, Gustave. *Études d'hygiène publique*. Paris and Nancy: Berger-Levrault, 1892.

———. *Législation des logements insalubres: Commentaires pratiques des lois du 15 février 1902 et du 7 avril 1903 relatives à la protection de la santé publique*. Paris: Berger-Levrault, 1904.

Kelsch, Louis-Félix-Achille. "Quelques réflexions sur la pathogénie des affections tuberculeuses, d'après observations cliniques et anatomo-pathologiques." Reprint of a paper given at the Academy of Medicine, February 7, 1893.

———. "Quelques réflexions sur la pathogénie et la prophylaxie de la tuberculose." *Bulletin médical*, June 17, 1908.

———. *Traité des maladies épidémiques: Étiologie et pathogénie des maladies infectieuses*. Paris: O. Doin, 1894.

Lépine, Louis, et al. "Notes générales de police: Organisation de la Police en France-Police administratif." In *Répertoire du droit administratif*, edited by M. E. Laferrière, vol. 22. Paris: Paul Dupont, 1905.

Locke, John. *An Essay Concerning Human Understanding*. London: Ward, Locke, and Co., 1881.

Monin, E. *Actualités d'hygiène et de médecine sociale: La Lutte pour la santé*. Paris: E. Flammarion, 1892.

Monod, Henri. *Le Choléra: Histoire d'une épidémie: Finistère, 1885–6.* Paris: Hachette, 1892.

———. *La Santé publique.* Paris: Hachette, 1904.

Ollivier, Auguste. *Études d'hygiène publique.* 4 vols. Paris: G. Steinheil, 1886–93.

Préfecture de Police. "Note en réponse au mémoire de M. le Préfet de la Seine sur les attributions de la Préfecture de Police." Paris, April 1858.

———. (E. Camescasse, préfet de police). "Rapport à Messieurs les Ministres de l'Intérieur et du Commerce, sur les mesures prises contre l'épidémie cholérique de 1884 à Paris et dans le département de la Seine." Paris: Chaix, 1885.

Préfecture de la Seine. (J. Bertillon, chef). "Tableaux statistiques de l'épidémie cholérique de 1884 à Paris et étude statistique des épidémies antérieurs." Service de la statistique municipale, Paris, 1886.

*Rapport sur la marche et les effets du choléra-morbus dans Paris et les communes rurales du Département de la Seine.* Paris: Imp. Nationale, 1834.

Rochard, Jules. "L'Avenir de l'hygiène." Paper given at the Association française pour l'avancement des sciences, Paris, 1887.

Rousseau, Jean-Jacques. *The Social Contract and Discourse on the Origin of Inequality,* edited by Lester G. Crocker. New York: Washington Square Press, 1967.

Sourdillon, Louis. *L'Autonomie communale à Paris et l'organisation administrative du département de la Seine.* Paris: Garnier frères, 1890.

Strauss, Paul. *La Croisade sanitaire.* Paris: E. Fasquell, 1902.

Strauss, Paul, and Alfred Fillassier. *Loi sur la protection de la santé publique (Loi du 15 février 1902): Travaux législatifs, guide pratique et commentaire.* 2d ed. Paris: J. Rousset, 1905.

Thoinot, Léon. *Histoire de l'épidémie cholérique de 1884: Origine-marche-étiologie générale.* Paris: G. Steinheil, 1885.

Tréhu, Émile. *Des pouvoirs de la municipalité parisienne en matière d'assainissement, l'application de la loi du 10 juillet 1894 sur l'assainissement de Paris et de la Seine.* Paris: Giard et E. Brière, 1905.

Villermé, Louis-René. *Tableau de l'état physique et moral des ouvriers employés dans les manufactures de coton, de laine et de soie.* 2 vols. Paris: Renouard, 1840.

Voltaire [François Marie Arouet]. *Philosophical Letters.* New York: Macmillan, 1961.

ARCHIVAL MATERIALS

National Archives (AN): C 3310, 3385, 5486, 5497, 5660; F[8] 171, 172, 208, 211, 212, 213.

Archives of the Prefecture of Police (APP): BA 307; DA 36, 304, 305, 306, 308, 309, 310, 311, 312, 313, 314; DB 454, 457, 458, 459.

Archives of the Prefecture of the Seine (AS): V$^{bis}$ 1I$^5$ 1; V$^{bis}$ 5.I$^5$ 1; V $^{bis}$ 5.I$^5$ 2; V$^{bis}$ 5$^1$ 5$^2$ ; VD$^6$370; VD$^6$ 779; VD$^6$ 780 1; VD$^6$ 1234; VD$^6$ 1344; VD$^6$ 1345; VD$^6$ 1347; V$^{bis}$ 4I$^5$ 3; V$^{bis}$ 4I$^5$ 4; V$^{bis}$ 15 15$^1$; V$^{bis}$ 15 I$^5$ 3; V$^{bis}$ 15 I$^5$ 4.

JOURNALS

*Annales d'hygiène publique et de médecine légale*
*Bulletin de l'Académie de médecine*
*Journal officiel: Débats parlementaires, Sénat*
*Journal officiel: Débats parlementaires, Chambre des députés*
*Moniteur universel*
*Revue d'hygiène*

*Secondary Sources*

Accampo, Elinor, Rachel G. Fuchs, and Mary Lynn Stewart. *Gender and the Politics of Social Reform in France, 1870–1914.* Baltimore: Johns Hopkins University Press, 1995.

Ackerknecht, Erwin. "Anticontagionism Between 1821 and 1867." *Bulletin of the History of Medicine* 22, no. 5 (1948): 562–93.

———. "Broussais, or a Forgotten Medical Revolution." *Bulletin of the History of Medicine* 27 (1953): 320–43.

———. "Hygiene in France, 1815–1848." *Bulletin of the History of Medicine* 22, no. 2 (1948): 117–55.

———. *Medicine at the Paris Hospital, 1794–1848.* Baltimore: Johns Hopkins University Press, 1967.

Aguet, J. P. *Les Grèves sous la monarchie de juillet (1830–1847): Contribution à l'étude du mouvement ouvrier français.* Geneva: Librarie E. Droz, 1954.

Aisenberg, Andrew R. "Contagious Disease and Urban Government in the Age of Pasteur." Ph.D. diss., Yale University, 1993.

Agulhon, Maurice. *La République au village.* Paris: Mouton, 1970.

———. *1848 ou l'apprentissage de la république.* Paris: Seuil, 1973.

Amann, Peter. *Revolution and Mass Democracy: The Paris Club Movement in 1848.* Princeton: Princeton University Press, 1975.

Baker, Keith Michael. "Closing the French Revolution: St. Simon and Comte." In *The Creation of Political Culture,* vol. 3: *The Transformation of Political Culture, 1789–1848,* edited by F. Furet and M. Ozouf, 323–39. Oxford: Pergamon Press, 1989.

———. *Condorcet: From Natural Philosophy to Social Mathematics.* Chicago: University of Chicago Press, 1975.

———. "Science and Politics at the End of the Old Regime." In *Inventing the French Revolution: Essays on French Political Culture in the Eighteenth Century,* 153–66. Cambridge: Cambridge University Press, 1990.

Barrows, Susanna. *Distorting Mirrors: Visions of the Crowd in Late Nineteenth-Century France*. New Haven: Yale University Press, 1981.

Berlière, Jean-Marc. *La Police des moeurs sous la IIIème République*. Paris: Seuil, 1992.

Bezucha, Robert. *The Lyon Uprising of 1834: Social and Political Conflict in a Nineteenth-Century City*. Cambridge: Harvard University Press, 1974.

Bono, James. "Science, Discourse, and Literature: The Role/Rule of Metaphor in Science." In *Literature and Science: Theory and Practice*, edited by Stuart Peterfreund, 59–89. Boston: Northeastern University Press, 1990.

———. *The Word of God and the Languages of Man: Interpreting Nature in Early Modern Science and Medicine*, vol. 1: *Ficino to Descartes*. Madison: University of Wisconsin Press, 1995.

Bourdelais, Patrice, and Jean-Yves Raulot. *Une Peur bleue: Histoire du choléra en France, 1832–54*. Paris: Payot, 1987.

Canguilhem, Georges. *Études d'histoire et de philosophie des sciences*. Paris: Vrin, 1989.

———. *Le Normal et le pathologique*. Paris: Presses universitaires, 1988.

———. "Puissance et limites de la rationalité en médecine." In *Médecine science et technique: Recueil d'études rédigées à l'occasion du centenaire de la mort de Claude Bernard (1813–1878)*, edited by Charles Marx, 109–30. Paris: CNRS, 1984.

Chevalier, Louis, ed. *Le Choléra: La Première épidémie du XIXème siècle*. La Roche-sur-Yon: Imp. centrale de l'Ouest, 1958.

———. *Laboring Classes and Dangerous Classes in Paris During the First Half of the Nineteenth Century*. Translated by Frank Jellinek. Princeton: Princeton University Press, 1973.

Clark, T. J. *The Painting of Modern Life: Paris in the Art of Manet and His Followers*. Princeton: Princeton University Press, 1984.

Coffin, Judith. "Social Science Meets Sweated Labor: Reinterpreting Women's Work in Late Nineteenth-Century France." *Journal of Modern History* 63 (June 1991): 230–70.

Cole, Joshua Hamilton. "The Power of Large Numbers: Population and Politics in Nineteenth-Century France." Ph.D. diss., University of California (Berkeley), 1991.

Coleman, William. *Death Is a Social Disease: Public Health and Political Economy in Early Industrial France*. Madison: University of Wisconsin Press, 1982.

Conry, Yvette. "Le 'Point de vue' de la médecine expérimentale selon Claude Bernard: Une Utopie positive?" In *Médecine science et technique: Recueil d'études rédigées à l'occasion du centenaire de la mort de Claude Bernard (1813–1878)*, edited by Charles Marx, 17–38. Paris: CNRS, 1984.

Cooter, Roger. "Anticontagionism and History's Medical Record." In *The*

*Problem of Medical Knowledge: Examining the Social Construction of Medicine*, edited by P. Wright and A. Treacher, 87–108. Edinburgh: Edinburgh University Press, 1982.

Corbin, Alain. *The Foul and the Fragrant: Odor and the French Social Imagination*. Translated by Miriam L. Kochan, with Dr. Roy Porter and Christopher Prendergast. Cambridge: Harvard University Press, 1986.

———. *Women for Hire: Prostitution and Sexuality in France After 1850*. Translated by Alan Sheridan. Cambridge: Cambridge University Press, 1990.

Dagognet, François. *Méthodes et doctrines dans l'oeuvre de Pasteur*. Paris: Press universitaires, 1967.

Darmon, Pierre. *La Longue traque de la variole*. Paris: Perrin, 1986.

De Kruif, Paul. *Microbe Hunters*. New York: Harcourt Brace, 1926.

Delaporte, François. *Disease and Civilization: The Cholera in Paris, 1832*. Translated by Arthur Goldhammer. Cambridge: MIT Press, 1986.

Dobo, Dr. Nicholas, and Dr. André Role. *Bichat: La Vie fulgurante d'un génie*. Paris: Perrin, 1989.

Donzelot, Jacques. *L'Invention du social: Essai sur le déclin des passions politiques*. Paris: Fayard, 1984.

———. *The Policing of Families*. Translated by Robert Hurley. New York: Pantheon, 1979.

Dubos, René. *Louis Pasteur: Free Lance of Science*. Boston: Little, Brown, 1950.

Ellis, Jack D. *The Physician-legislators: Medicine and Politics in the Early Third Republic, 1870–1914*. Cambridge: Cambridge University Press, 1990.

Elwitt, Sanford. *The Making of the Third Republic: Class and Politics in France, 1868–1884*. Baton Rouge: Louisiana State University Press, 1975.

———. *The Third Republic Defended: Bourgeois Reform in France, 1880–1914*. Baton Rouge: Louisiana State University Press, 1986.

Engelstein, Laura. *The Keys to Happiness: Sex and the Search for Modernity in Fin-de-Siècle Russia*. Ithaca: Cornell University Press, 1992.

Epstein, Steven. *Impure Science: AIDS, Activism, and the Politics of Knowledge*. Berkeley: University of California Press, 1996.

Evans, Richard J. *Death in Hamburg: Society and Politics in the Cholera Years, 1830–1910*. London: Oxford University Press, 1987.

Ewald, François. *L'État providence*. Paris: Grasset, 1986.

Faure, Alain. "Classe malpropre, classe dangereuse? Quelques remarques à propos des chiffonniers parisiens au XIXᵉ siècle et leurs cités." *Recherches* 29 (1978): 79–102.

Foucault, Michel. *The Birth of the Clinic: An Archaeology of Medical Perception*. Translated by A. M. Sheridan. New York: Vintage Books, 1975.

————. *Discipline and Punish: The Birth of the Prison.* Translated by A. M. Sheridan. New York: Pantheon Books, 1973.

————. "Governmentality." In *The Foucault Effect,* edited by Graham Burchell, Colin Gordon, and Peter Miller, 87–104. Chicago: University of Chicago Press, 1991.

————. *The History of Sexuality,* vol. 1: *An Introduction.* New York: Vintage Books, 1980.

————. *The Order of Things: An Archaeology of the Human Sciences.* New York: Vintage Books, 1973.

————, ed. *Politiques de l'habitat, 1800–50.* Paris: Collège de France, Comité de la recherche et du développement en architecture, 1977.

Fraisse, Geneviève. *Reason's Muse: Sexual Difference and the Birth of Democracy.* Trans. Jane Marie Todd. Chicago: University of Chicago Press, 1994.

Gaillard, Jeanne. "Assistance et urbanisme dans le Paris du Second Empire." In *L'Haleine des faubourgs: Ville, habitat et santé au xixème siècle,* edited by Lion Murard and Patrick Zylberman, 395–422. Fontenay-sous-Bois: Recherches, 1978.

————. *Paris, la ville (1852–1870).* Paris: Honoré Champion, 1977.

Geison, Gerald L. "Pasteur." In *Dictionary of Scientific Biography,* vol. 10, edited by Charles Coulston Gillispie, 350–416. New York: Charles Scribner's Sons, 1974.

————. *The Private Science of Louis Pasteur.* Princeton: Princeton University Press, 1995.

Giddens, Anthony, ed. *Durkheim on Politics and the State.* Stanford: Stanford University Press, 1986.

Gillispie, Charles Coulston. *Science and Polity in France at the End of the Old Regime.* Princeton: Princeton University Press, 1980.

Goldstein, Jan. *Console and Classify: The French Psychiatric Profession in the Nineteenth Century.* Cambridge: Cambridge University Press, 1987.

————. "'Moral Contagion': A Professional Ideology of Medicine and Psychiatry in Eighteenth- and Nineteenth-Century France." In *Professions and the French State, 1700–1900,* edited by Gerald Geison, 181–222. Philadelphia: University of Pennsylvania Press, 1984.

Gossez, Rémi. *Les Ouvriers de Paris,* vol. 1: *L'Organisation, 1848–1851.* Bibliothèque de la Révolution de 1848., vol. 24: La Roche-sur-Yon: Imprimerie centrale de l'Ouest, 1967.

Grmek, M. D. "La Conception de la maladie et de la santé chez Claude Bernard." In *L'Aventure de la science: Mélanges Alexandre Koyré,* 208–27. Paris: Hermann, 1964.

Guerrand, Roger-Henri. "La Bataille du tout-à-l'égout." *L'Histoire* 53 (February 1983): 66–74.

Gusdorf, Georges. *Les Sciences humaines et la pensée occidentale,* vol. 8: *La Conscience révolutionnaire: Les idéologues.* Paris: Payot, 1978.

Hacking, Ian. *The Taming of Chance.* Cambridge: Cambridge University Press, 1990.

Hanaway, Caroline. "Medicine, Public Welfare and the State in Eighteenth-Century France: The Société royale de médecine de Paris, 1776–1793." Ph.D. diss., Johns Hopkins University, 1974.

Haraway, Donna. *Primate Visions: Gender, Race, and Nature in the World of Modern Science.* New York: Routledge, 1989.

Hatzfeld, Henri. *Du paupérisme à la sécurité sociale, 1850–1914.* Paris: Armand Colin, 1971.

Hayward, J. E. S. "The Official Social Philosophy of the French Third Republic: Léon Bourgeois and Solidarism." *International Review of Social History* 6 (1961): 19–48.

Heilbroner, Robert L., ed. *The Essential Adam Smith.* New York: W. W. Norton, 1986.

Holmes, Frederic L. *Claude Bernard and Animal Chemistry: The Emergence of a Scientist.* Cambridge: Harvard University Press, 1974.

Jacquemet, Gérard. "Urbanisme parisien: La Bataille du tout-à-l'égout à la fin du dix-neuvième siècle." *Revue d'histoire moderne et contemporaine* 26 (October–December 1979): 505–48.

Jones, H. S. *The French State in Question: Public Law and Political Argument in the Third Republic.* Cambridge: Cambridge University Press, 1993.

Jordan, David P. *Transforming Paris: The Life and Labors of Baron Haussmann.* New York: Free Press, 1995.

Krüger, Lorenz, Lorraine Daston, and Michael Heidelberger, eds. *The Probabilistic Revolution,* vol. 2: *Ideas in History.* Cambridge: MIT Press, 1987.

Kudlick, Catherine J. *Cholera in Post-Revolutionary Paris: A Cultural History.* Berkeley: University of California Press, 1986.

La Berge, Ann F. *Mission and Method: The Early Nineteenth-century French Public Health Movement.* Cambridge: Cambridge University Press, 1992.

Latour, Bruno. *Les Microbes: Guerre et paix; suivi de irréductions.* Paris: Métailié, 1984.

———. "Pasteur et Pouchet: Hétérogenèse de l'histoire des sciences." In *Éléments d'histoire des sciences,* edited by Michel Serres, 423–45. Paris: Bordas, 1989.

———. *The Pasteurization of France.* Translated by Alan Sheridan and John Law. Cambridge: Harvard University Press, 1988.

———. *Science in Action: How to Follow Scientists and Engineers Through Society.* Cambridge: Harvard University Press, 1987.

Latour, Bruno, and Steve Woolgar. *Laboratory Life: The Social Construction of*

*Scientific Facts.* Princeton: Princeton University Press, 1986. (Originally published by Sage Publications, 1979.)

Léonard, Jacques. *Les Médecins de l'Ouest au XIX<sup>e</sup> siècle.* 3 vols. Paris: Honoré Champion, 1978.

Lesch, John. "The Paris Academy of Medicine and Experimental Science, 1820–1848." In *The Investigative Enterprise: Experimental Physiology in Nineteenth-Century Medicine,* edited by William Coleman and Frederic L. Holmes, 100–138. Berkeley: University of California Press, 1988.

———. *Science and Medicine in France: The Emergence of Experimental Physiology, 1790–1855.* Cambridge: Harvard University Press, 1984.

Lukes, Steven. *Émile Durkheim: His Life and Works.* Stanford: Stanford University Press, 1985.

Lynch, Katherine A. *Family, Class, and Ideology in Early Industrial France: Social Policy and the Working-Class Family, 1825–48.* Madison: University of Wisconsin Press, 1988.

Marcus, Sharon. *Apartment Stories: The City and the Home in Nineteenth-Century Paris and London.* Berkeley: University of California Press, 1998.

Margadant, Ted W. *French Peasants in Revolt: The Insurrection of 1851.* Princeton: Princeton University Press, 1979.

Maulitz, Russell C. *Morbid Appearances: The Anatomy of Pathology in the Early Nineteenth Century.* Cambridge: Cambridge University Press, 1987.

Merriman, John. *The Agony of the Republic: The Repression of the Left in Revolutionary France, 1848–51.* New Haven: Yale University Press, 1978.

Mitchell, Allan. *The Divided Path: The German Influence on Social Reform in France After 1870.* Chapel Hill: University of North Carolina Press, 1991.

Moulin, A. M. "The Pasteur Institutes Between the Two World Wars: The Shuffling of the International Sanitary Order." In *International Health Organizations and Movements, 1918–39,* edited by P. Weindling, 244–65. Cambridge: Cambridge University Press, 1995.

———. "Patriarchal Science: The Network of the Overseas Pasteur Institutes." In *Science and Empires: Historical Studies About Scientific Development and European Expansion,* edited by C. Jami, A. M. Moulin, and P. Petitjean, 307–22. Dordrecht: Kluwer, 1992.

Murard, Lion, and Patrick Zylberman. *L'Hygiène dans la république: La Santé publique en France, ou l'utopie contrariée, 1870–1918.* Paris: Fayard, 1996.

Murphy, Terrence D. "Medical Knowledge and Statistical Methods in Early Nineteenth-Century France." *Medical History* 25 (1981): 301–19.

Nicolet, Claude. *L'Idée républicaine en France: Essai d'histoire critique, 1789–1924.* Paris: Gallimard, 1982.

Nord, Philip. *The Republican Moment: Struggles for Democracy in Nineteenth-Century France.* Cambridge: Harvard University Press, 1995.

Nye, Robert. *Crime, Madness, and Politics in Modern France: The Medical Concept of National Decline*. Princeton: Princeton University Press, 1984.

O'Brien, Patricia. *The Promise of Punishment: Prisons in Nineteenth-Century France*. Princeton: Princeton University Press, 1982.

———. "Urban Growth and Public Order: The Development of a Modern Police in Paris, 1829–1854." Ph.D. diss., Columbia University, 1973.

Olmsted, J. M. D., and E. H. Olmsted. *Claude Bernard and the Experimental Method*. New York: Henry Schumann, 1952.

Osborne, Michael A. "French Military Epidemiology and the Limits of the Laboratory: The Case of Louis-Félix-Achille Kelsch." In *The Laboratory Revolution in Medicine*, edited by Andrew Cunningham and Perry Williams, 189–208. Cambridge: Cambridge University Press, 1992.

Pedersen, Susan. *Family, Dependence, and the Origins of the Welfare State in Britain and France, 1914–45*. Cambridge: Cambridge University Press, 1993.

Pelling, Margaret. *Cholera, Fever and English Medicine, 1825–1865*. Oxford: Oxford University Press, 1978.

Perrot, Michelle. "On the Fringe." In *From the Fires of Revolution to the Great War*, edited by Michelle Perrot, 241–59. Vol 4 of *A History of Private Life*, edited by Philippe Ariès and Georges Duby. Cambridge: Belknap Press of Harvard University Press, 1990.

Pinkney, David H. *The French Revolution of 1830*. Princeton: Princeton University Press, 1982.

———. *Napoleon III and the Rebuilding of Paris*. Princeton: Princeton University Press, 1958.

Poovey, Mary. *Making a Social Body: British Cultural Formation, 1830–1864*. Chicago: University of Chicago Press, 1995.

Poupa, Otakar. "Le Problème de l'évolution chez Claude Bernard." In *Philosophie et méthodologie scientifiques de Claude Bernard*, edited by Etienne Wolff et al., 109–16. Paris: Masson, 1967.

Price, Roger. *The French Second Republic: A Social History*. Ithaca: Cornell University Press, 1972.

Procacci, Giovanna. *Gouverner la misère: La Question sociale en France, 1789–1848*. Paris: Seuil, 1993.

———. "Sociology and Its Poor." *Politics and Society* 17 (1989): 163–87.

Ramsey, Matthew. "Public Health in France." In *The History of Public Health and the Modern State*, edited by Dorothy Porter, 45–118. Amsterdam: Clio Medica, 1994.

Ratcliffe, Barrie. "Perception and Realities of the Urban Margin: The Rag Pickers of Paris in the First Half of the Nineteenth Century." *Canadian Journal of History/Annales canadiennes d'histoire* 27 (August 1992): 198–233.

Reddy, William. *The Rise of Market Culture: The Textile Trade and French Society, 1750–1900*. Cambridge: Cambridge University Press, 1984.

Reid, Donald. *Paris Sewers and Sewermen: Realities and Representations*. Cambridge: Harvard University Press, 1991.

Rigaudias-Weiss, Hilde. *Les Enquêtes ouvrières en France*. Paris: Presses universitaires, 1936. Reprint, New York: Arno Press, 1975.

Riley, Denise. *"Am I That Name"?: Feminism and the Category of "Women" in History*. London: Macmillan, 1988.

Rosanvallon, Pierre. *L'État en France de 1789 à nos jours*. Paris: Seuil, 1990.

Rosen, George. "Cameralism and the Concept of Medical Police." *Bulletin of the History of Medicine* 27 (1953): 21–42.

Sauvy, Alfred. *Histoire économique de la France entre les deux guerres*. 4 vols. Paris: Fayard, 1965–70.

Schafer, Sylvia. *Children in Moral Danger and the Problem of Government in Third Republic France*. Princeton: Princeton University Press, 1997.

Schiller, Joseph. *Claude Bernard et les problèmes scientifiques de son temps*. Paris: Editions du cèdre, 1967.

Scott, Joan Wallach. *Gender and the Politics of History*. New York: Columbia University Press, 1988.

———. *Only Paradoxes to Offer: French Feminists and the Rights of Man*. Cambridge: Harvard University Press, 1996.

Sewell, William. *Work and Revolution in France: The Language of Labor from the Revolution to 1848*. Cambridge: Cambridge University Press, 1980.

Shapin, Steven, and Simon Schaffer. *Leviathan and the Air-Pump: Hobbes, Boyle, and the Experimental Life*. Princeton: Princeton University Press, 1985.

Shapiro, Ann-Louise. *Breaking the Codes: Female Criminality in Fin-de-Siècle Paris*. Stanford: Stanford University Press, 1996.

———. *Housing the Poor of Paris, 1850–1902*. Madison: University of Wisconsin Press, 1985.

Shinn, Terry. *L'École polytechnique, 1794–1914*. Paris: Presses de la Fondation nationale des sciences politiques, 1980.

Snowden, Frank M. *Naples in the Time of Cholera, 1884–1911*. Cambridge: Cambridge University Press, 1995.

Salomon-Bayet, Claire, ed. *Pasteur et la révolution pastorienne*. Paris: Payot, 1986.

Staum, Martin S. *Cabanis: Enlightenment and Medical Philosophy in the French Revolution*. Princeton: Princeton University Press, 1980.

Stone, Judith F. *The Search for Social Peace: Reform Legislation in France, 1890–1914*. Albany: State University of New York Press, 1985.

Sussman, George D. "From Yellow Fever to Cholera: A Study of French Government Policy, Medical Professionalism and Popular Movements in the Epidemic Crises of the Restoration and the July Monarchy." Ph.D. diss., Yale University, 1971.

Sutcliffe, Anthony. *The Autumn of Central Paris: The Defeat of Town Planning, 1850–1870*. London: Edward Arnold, 1970.

Tilly, Charles. *The Contentious French*. Cambridge: Belknap Press of Harvard University Press, 1985.

———. "Did the Cake of Custom Break?" In *Consciousness and Class Experience*, edited by John M. Merriman, 17–44. New York: Holmes and Meier, 1979.

Tilly, Charles, and Lynn Lees. "Le Peuple de juin 1848." *Annales E.S.C.* 29 (September–October 1974): 1061–91.

Weber, Eugen. *Peasants into Frenchmen: The Modernization of Rural France, 1870–1914*. Stanford: Stanford University Press, 1976.

Weisz, George. *The Medical Mandarins: The French Academy of Medicine in the Nineteenth and Early Twentieth Centuries*. Oxford: Oxford University Press, 1995.

Williams, Elizabeth A. *The Physical and the Moral: Anthropology, Physiology, and Philosophical Medicine in France, 1750–1850*. Cambridge: Cambridge University Press, 1994.

Wohl, Robert. *French Communism in the Making, 1914–1924*. Stanford: Stanford University Press, 1966.

# Index

In this index an "f" after a number indicates a separate reference on the next page, and an "ff" indicates separate references on the next two pages. A continuous discussion over two or more pages is indicated by a span of page numbers, e.g., "57–59." *Passim* is used for a cluster of references in close but not consecutive sequence.

hygiene commissions, 158–61; early uses of the term, 158f; and conditions of the home, 159, 163; process of discovering and regulating the, 167–76. *See also* working-class dwelling

Franche-comté, 71

François Miron, rue, 127, 145

Franco-Prussian War, 58, 87, 98; populationist debate in wake of 130; morbidity and mortality statistics for disease during the, 130

Frégier, Honoré, 34, 41–45, 128; reference to contagion in work of, 42ff

Fuilhan, M., 145

Gaffky, Georg, 78

Garet, Maurice, 209n72

*garnis*, 115, 120, 137

Geison, Gerald, 75, 196n31

Gendron, M., 145

Gennevilliers, 106–10 *passim*

Gentilly, 22

germs, theory of (Pasteur), 71. *See also* debate over contagion

Gibert, Joseph, 92

Girard, M., 110

Gironde (department of the), 51

glanders, 68f, 77

government regulation: limited by Republican legacy of rights, 2, 44f, 138, 142f; justified by contagion, 3f, 11, 25–32 *passim*, 38, 41f; and science, 4–12 *passim*, 18, 32, 40, 179; role reassessed in light of Paris Commune of 1871, 58–65; in debate over contagion, 67, 70f, 76, 81f; in Bouchard's understanding of contagion, 84; in Michel Peter's understanding of contagion, 87; and "New Hygiene," 87–94 *passim*, 99, 103f; expanded through establishment of Bureau des épidémies, 117, 121, 123; expansion in the home justified by danger of the foyer, 128, 165; in debates for a public health law, 131; and neighborhood hygiene commissions, 145f, 150, 153f. *See also* science

Grancher, Joseph, 80

*grands boulevards*, 60

Granger, M., 169

Guéneau de Mussy, François, 69ff

Guérin, Jules, 68f, 125

Hardy, Dr., 125

Haussmann, Georges: career of, 51; reliance on 1850 Insalubrious Dwellings Law, 51f; and expansion of attributions of Prefecture of the Seine, 51f, 111; demise in 1860s, 58

Haussmannization: and sewer system, 105f, 110f; criticized by hygienists, 113–15, 122f, 129, 148

Hébrard, M., 152

Hervieux, Jacques., 79

*Histoire de l'administration de la police de Paris depuis Philippe-Auguste jusqu'aux Etats généraux* (Honoré Frégier), 43ff

*Histoire des sciences médicales* (Charles Daremberg), 142

home, *see* working-class dwelling

Hôpital Enfant Jésus, 80

hospitals: and cholera epidemic of 1832, 16; and question of microbial transmission, 81; as source of information for understanding contagion, 91, 158; and isolation techniques, 141

Hôtel Dieu, 16

hygiene: in Cabanis' work, 9; and investigation of social problems, 27, 30; in 1850 Insalubrious Dwellings Law, 48; and regulation of prostitution, 59f; reinvigorated around microbial cause of disease, 84, 87–89, 98f; as superior form of scientific observation, 96, 101. *See also* hygienists

hygienists: contribution to understandings of contagion, 4f; professional strategies of, 10, 88–93 *passim*, 101, 103, 111f, 117, 123, 129, 134f; support of social legislation, 10, 112; and miasmatic theory of disease, 21; and prison regulation, 43; in conflict with engineers over *tout-à-l'égout*, 105–12; as ex-

Library of Congress Cataloging-in-Publication Data

Aisenberg, Andrew Robert.
  Contagion : disease, government, and the "social question" in
nineteenth-century France / Andrew R. Aisenberg.
    p.   cm.
  Includes bibliographical references and index.
  ISBN 0-8047-3395-3 (cloth : alk. paper)
    1. Communicable diseases—Social aspects—France—History—
19th century.  2. Communicable diseases—Political aspects—
France—History—19th century.  3. Communicable diseases—
France—Social policy—History—19th century.  4. Medicine—
Social aspects—France—History—19th century.  5. Medicine—
Political aspects—France—History—19th century.  6. Medical
care—Social aspects—France—History—19th century.  7. Medical
care—Political aspects—France—History—19th century.  8. Health
reformers—France—History—19th century.  9. France—Social
conditions—History—19th century.  I. Title.

RA643.7.F8A37    1999
306.4'.61'094409034—dc21                                    98-36505
                                                                CIP


Original printing 1999
Last figure below indicates year of this printing:
08   07   06   05   04   03   02   01   00   99